CONNECTIVE TISSUE MANIPULATIONS

This volume represents the third and extended edition of the book "Connective Tissue Massage."

CONNECTIVE TISSUE MANIPULATIONS

THEORY AND THERAPEUTIC APPLICATION

BY

MARIA EBNER

F.C.S.P. (Dip. T.P.); Diploma in Physical Education (Vienna University); former Principal of School and Department of Physiotherapy of the United Leeds Hospitals

KRIEGER PUBLISHING COMPANY
MALABAR, FLORIDA

Original Edition 1985
Prior edition appeared under the title
"Connective Tissue Massage"

Printed and Published by
ROBERT E. KRIEGER PUBLISHING CO., INC.
KRIEGER DRIVE
MALABAR, FL 32950

Printed in the United States of America.

Library of Congress Cataloging in Publication Data

Ebner, Maria.
Connective tissue manipulations.

Rev. ed. of: Connective tissue massage. 1975, c1962.
Includes index.
1. Massage. 2. Connective tissues. I. Ebner, Maria. Connective tissue massage. II. Title.
[DNLM: 1. Connective Tissue. 2. Massage. WB 537 E16c]
RM721.E35 1985 615.8'22 84-9636
ISBN 0-89874-763-5

10 9 8 7

Preface to Third Edition

This book was originally written to provide a well illustrated help for the Therapist who wished to learn a new technique which also represented a new approach to the patient. It still continues to fulfill this purpose. The second revised Edition, which changed its publication from Great Britain to America, was able to add an account of the experience gained during Lecture Tours in many parts of the world and the extended use and adaptation for effective use of C.T.M. in a number of conditions where previously very little help had been available with conventional Drug or other Therapy.

The generous offer of the Publishers to put into print the development and experience of research in Medical and Allied Sciences by members of the Medical and Allied Professions has led to the publication of a third and extended and revised edition. The result of the global approach to the patient has extended the use of the technique into new fields such as Psychiatry and Sports Medicine. The exciting Research Publications of the Department of Dermatology of Vienna University will eventually lead to a better understanding of recovery processes and the role C.T.M. can play in them.

My personal gratitude is therefore particularly due to Professor Niebauer of Vienna University, Dr. A. McKechnie, Consultant of Bangour Village Hospital and many Physiotherapy Colleagues, particular gratitude is due to the teaching efforts of Miss Nan Watson, Superintendent Physiotherapist.

Last but not least I should like to thank the Publishers for their generous offer of publication during a universally difficult economical situation.

Southport,1984 M.E.

Preface to Second Edition

Since the last Edition, I have been fortunate in having been able to follow invitations for Lecture Tours and Clinical Teaching in South Africa, New Zealand, Australia, New York and Canada in addition to numerous courses in Great Britain. The clinical experience gained by the treatment of a great variety of patients by myself and a number of my colleagues has made it possible to describe the effects of Connective Tissue Massage more clearly and appreciate the effects of this treatment in a number of conditions where little help could be given up to now both by Drug-Therapy as well as Physiotherapy without causing detrimental Side-effects. I should like to mention in particular conditions such as Scleroderma, Migraine and Intermittent Claudication. In particular I should like to thank my colleagues Miss Nan Watson from Bangour General Hospital, Miss Adaline Sellar from Mearnskirk Hospital and Mrs. E. N. Cook from Ottawa and the Consultant Surgeons and Physicians from these hospitals whose interest made this treatment available to patients.

I hope that this new revised edition will help to make the Physiotherapist's work more effective and help the doctor appreciate the clinical situation more clearly and therefore give the physiotherapist more effective guidance. Unfortunately there are still not sufficient research results available to explain factually all the beneficial clinical results. Some research projects which are carried out at present may help in the future to add factual knowledge to intelligent reasoning.

All members of the Medical and Para-Medical professions are continuously concerned to find new ways to help patients to return again to a fuller and therefore more satisfying life. I therefore hope that this new edition will not only allow me to address a wider audience but make literature again available to doctors and colleagues.

I therefore would finally like to thank the Publishers who by their cooperation during difficult times have made this revised Edition possible.

Leeds, 1974. M. E.

Preface to First Edition

I SHOULD like to express my gratitude to the Board of Governors of the United Leeds Hospitals who granted leave of absence so that I should be able to attend a course on Connective Tissue Massage arranged by Professor Kohlrausch in Hamburg in 1954. The excellent teaching of this well-known German physician made it possible to carry out on my return, with the authority of a number of consultants, experimental treatments. These produced very gratifying results. A second visit to Germany in 1958 to attend a course arranged by Dr Teirich-Leube in Freiburg im Breisgau gave further opportunity to gain knowledge in a subject which is taught in most Physiotherapy Schools in Germany and practised in a number of European countries.

It has been my privilege to arrange a number of post-graduate courses in England, Scotland and Ireland for physiotherapists who were anxious to learn new methods of treatment. It became clear that a reference book in English was needed for use after the courses. These courses would not have been possible without the generous help given by a number of medical consultants. To them and in particular to Professor S. J. Hartfall, Consultant Physician at the General Infirmary, Leeds, I should like to express my gratitude for their interest and encouragement.

I am indebted to my colleagues, especially to Miss Ruth Nicholl, who by their loyal co-operation made the collection of many detailed case histories possible. I must also express my grateful appreciation to Miss M. D. Brown, Medical Artist at the University of Leeds, who changed my rough sketches into clear and delightful diagrams. Thanks are also due to the Department of Medical Photography of the General Infirmary at Leeds for the excellent photographic illustrations.

Finally, I should like to thank most sincerely the publishers for their unfailing help and co-operation in the publication of a book on a new subject.

M. E.

LEEDS, 1962.

Contents

Introduction

When approaching the subject of connective tissue massage it is very important not to compare it with the more conventional forms of massage at present used in the countries of the British Commonwealth. The results obtained with this conventional massage can be explained comparatively satisfactorily. Mennell's statement (1945) that there are two, and only two, possible effects of any movement of massage is still true. They are *reflex* and *mechanical.*

When finally persuaded by English colleagues to write a book on connective tissue massage I was fully aware of the many difficulties which would have to be overcome. These difficulties are not confined to those facing every author writing a textbook on a special technique but are increased in this case by the fact that a number of the effects obtained by this specialized technique cannot be explained satisfactorily in the light of available knowledge. In the beginning this technique was mainly used on patients referred by doctors because other forms of therapy had proved unsatisfactory. Gradually patients were selected carefully, taking into consideration satisfactory results obtained in previous cases. These results, which have frequently helped patients to return to a useful life, have encouraged me to undertake the revision of a book which I hope will prove helpful to others. It is intended to give written information which will amplify the knowledge gained in courses. It might be necessary later to modify some of the explanations given on the effects of the massage; it has proved advisable since the last Edition to modify some details of treatment in the light of past experience taking into consideration anatomical and physiological facts. This applies particularly to the use of short and long strokes, connections of superficial muscles such as Latissimus Dorsi and to rest-periods after treatment. The most important information which has been gained since the last Edition is due to the development of Electromicroscopy in the research work carried out at the Universities of Innsbruck and Vienna in Austria and in particular by Professor Niebauer and al. The literature can be found under "References". Further clinical experience and the knowledge gained by research in the basic sciences has encouraged Medical Consultants and Physiotherapists working with them to extend the use of C.T.M. further afield. Some of Professor Niebauer's work will be referred to in the Chapter III on Skin. Completely new therapeutic fields have been entered by using C.T.M. in Psychiatry and Sports Medicine and the use of the technique has been further extended in the field of circulatory diseases. The clinical results obtained in the last 30 years amply justify any work which can make this form of therapy available to more patients. This is particularly important in an age where the dangers of Drug therapy have been recognised and the value of a global approach appreciated. The value of a personal therapeutic approach as compared to a computerised mechanical approach is also becoming obvious.

A textbook on any particular technique can never replace the practical learning of a skilled movement. It can, however, help to impart knowledge gained in past years of experience and study, which may help others to build on a sound basis and gain further insight into a subject which may help to restore patients to a fuller and happier life.

This type of massage was originated by Elisabeth Dicke of Germany who in 1929 suffered from a severe disturbance in the peripheral circulation of her right leg. As a result of a neglected tooth infection a general toxaemia had developed which resulted in an endarteritis obliterans of the right leg. This leg was cold and bluish in colour, the toes giving the appearance of incipient gangrene. The dorsalis pedis artery was no longer palpable. Frau Dicke was advised to consider amputation of the lower limb. In addition to the extreme pain in the extremity, she suffered from almost unbearable backache. While lying on her side she tried to give herself some relief by stroking over the painful areas of the back. She found that over the sacrum and over the right iliac crest thickenings and infiltrations could be palpated, while towards the left side on the same level the skin felt tight. She tried to ease the tension by stroking with the fingers across the affected areas. She found that these areas were hypersensitive to touch, slight stroking with the fingertip causing great pain. The tension, however, gradually subsided, the pain in the back eased and an agreeable sensation of warmth took its place. While persisting on successive days with the stroking pins and needles were gradually felt in the affected leg, followed by a sensation of warmth. In further treatments she incorporated the areas round the great trochanter and along the iliotibial tract. Gradually the superficial venous circulation reappeared in the thigh and leg. The severe symptoms subsided after a further three months' treatment carried out by a colleague under Frau Dicke's direction. She was able to resume her occupation as a physiotherapist after a year.

Years of investigation followed. During the course of her illness Frau Dicke had experienced pathological function of internal organs in addition to the symptoms in the back and leg. She suffered from a chronic gastritis, the liver showed enlargement, the heart showed symptoms of angina, and finally she experienced disturbance of kidney function. These visceral complaints cleared up simultaneously with the improvement of peripheral circulation and normalization of tissue changes in the back. Treatment of pathologically affected areas of the body surface helped to clear up pathological changes in affected viscera. She discovered that certain areas on the body surface definitely belonged to certain viscera. Systematic observation of patients during the course of the following years confirmed these findings. Unknown to her at the time the English neurologist, Head (1898), had already described similar findings of changes in well-defined areas of body surface pertaining invariably to certain organs. These alterations appear when pathological changes take place in affected viscera and are known in the literature as "Head's zones."

Further clinical investigations followed in 1935 under Professor Veil in Jena and in 1938 under Professor Kohlrausch and Dr Leube in Freiburg im Breisgau, incorporating also the basic work of Mackenzie. While Head pointed out changes in skin areas, Mackenzie (1917) drew attention to changes in muscle tone and sensitivity in areas which share the same root supply with pathologically affected organs.

Years of work and investigation resulted in the present-day method of Bindegewebsmassage in Germany, and this is used in most countries in Europe. The method is now widely employed not only in pathological conditions associated with visceral disease but in the treatment of diseases associated with pathology of circulation, in which it shows very gratifying results. In Germany it is also widely used by members of the medical profession for diagnostic purposes.

My own clinical experience has amply justified the claims made by German workers. Present-day knowledge seems to make it impossible to explain the results on a purely neurological reflex basis. An effort will be made in later chapters to give a reasoned account of the rationale of this type of treatment. The author is fully aware that it is impossible at the moment to account for all the effects on a scientific basis.

Head first drew attention to the fact that pathological changes in viscera are accompanied by changes in cutaneous areas supplied by the same root segments. Mackenzie (1917) pointed out changes in muscle tone in groups of muscles associated with the root supply of pathologically affected viscera. Frau Dicke's valuable contribution (1953) consists of her discovery that pathological alterations can also take place in subcutaneous tissue. Professor Niebauer and al. (1972, 1977) have carried out most important research about the structure and functions of the skin, in particular about its nerve supply and connections to other parts of the human organism and the presence of cells which probably have a trophic function.

The most superficial layer of the tissues forming the body surface is the skin. It represents the immediate link with the external environment. It contains the exteroreceptors, *i.e.*, specialized nerve endings which react to touch in various intensities and to changes in temperature such as heat and cold.* The deepest layer forming the body surface is that of the muscles. These again contain numerous nerve endings which can alter the tension in the tissue both reflexly and voluntarily. These nerve endings also register alterations in the tension of the tissue by means of proprioceptors, *i.e.,* specialized nerve endings sensitive to alterations in the length of the muscle fibre. Both these tissues link up with the somatic as well as the autonomic nervous system. This link-up will be responsible for vascular changes in both tissues. The layer of tissue between skin and muscle consists of connective tissue proper, and this is the layer of tissue which is particularly important for the massage manipulation discussed in this book. The state of tension in this tissue will primarily depend on its vascularity and the consistency of its blood supply.

The term "connective tissue massage" might indicate that the manipulation deals with the tissue as such. This is not quite correct. The manipulation takes place *in* the connective tissue layer, but it is not yet quite clear which elements present in this tissue receive effective stimuli. Therefore, as a more accurate term is not at present to hand, the term "connective tissue massage" has been retained.

*T.o.*American Osteopathic Ass.,* January 1955.

CHAPTER I

Connective Tissue—Anatomy and Function

CONNECTIVE tissue is present in the human body in two main varieties: (1) formed connective tissue, and (2) loose connective tissue. It is loose connective tissue which will have to be considered mainly for the purpose of this work. Loose connective tissue is very widely distributed in the human body. It forms the superficial and deep fascia, the intermuscular septa; it surrounds blood vessels and nerves and forms part of the framework of most organs. It provides a true connecting link between all structures and may be considered to pass like a spider's web through the body. Round muscles it forms the epimysial sheaths. It also forms the perivascular and perineural sheaths, the fibrous capsule for glands and organs. The superficial fascia supports nerves, blood vessels, lymphatics and sometimes muscles. Superficially it blends with the true cutis. Deep fascia surrounds muscle groups, attaches to bone and blends with the periosteum. In its areolar variety it forms tissue spaces.

ANATOMY OF LOOSE CONNECTIVE TISSUE

The development of all vertebrates, including human, begins with a sperm—fertilized egg—a single cell which soon divides into daughter cells. These continue to divide and soon begin to be arranged in three distinct layers which are called the fundamental germ layers. Their arrangement in the embryo is indicated by their names, *i.e.*, ectoderm (the outer layer), mesoderm (the middle layer) and entoderm (the inner layer). The cells of each layer continue to divide, differentiate and help to form specialized tissues. The mesodermal cell layers originally develop between ectodermal and entodermal cell layers, but soon push their way between the cell layers of ectoderm and entoderm. The tissues and structures derived from the mesoderm are: all connective and supporting tissue, lymphatic organs with very few exceptions, blood cells, bone marrow, skeletal, cardiac and smooth muscle with the exception of smooth muscle of sweat glands and pupillary muscle, the endothelial lining of blood and lymphatic vessels, the serous membranes of pleura, pericardium and peritoneum, the suprarenal cortex and part of the epithelial lining of the urinary system.

All varieties of connective tissue consist of cells and an intercellular substance or matrix. In connective tissue proper the intercellular substance, apart from the fibres, is soft.

Cell varieties occurring, and defined so far by various methods of investigation, are: the fibroblast or fixed connective tissue cell, histiocytes or macrophages, mast cells and wandering cells from the blood.

Many scientists consider that loose connective tissue is an undifferentiated form of embryonic connective tissue, which has many potentialities and can develop into many other forms of tissue. If it is distended with air or fluid it becomes evident that large numbers of spaces exist between the fibres. In these spaces is to be found the ground substance and tissue fluid. The tissue fluid represents material derived from the plasma. It holds the water-soluble proteins, crystaloids, metabolites and gases.

Fibroblasts are one of the two most numerous cell types of loose connective tissue. They are large, flat, branching cells with extensive processes which may touch the processes of other fibroblasts. The cell membrane is very delicate, the nucleus is oval or spherical and the cytoplasm is homogenous or finely granular. As their name suggests, they are concerned with the formation of fibres. Following trauma, these cells enlarge and become particularly active. Their function seems therefore to be primarily that of building.

Histiocytes are the second most numerous variety of loose connective tissue cells. They are irregularly shaped cells with processes which are usually short; the nucleus is often smaller than that of the fibroblast. In the resting state the cytoplasm contains some granules and vacuoles. Under healthy conditions these cells are probably quiescent, but become amoeboid and phagocytic under abnormal conditions such as inflammation. Their function seems therefore to be primarily the function of scavengers.

The plasma cells are comparatively small in number. They are smaller than the histiocytes, and are of ovoid or irregular shape with a homogenous cytoplasm. The nucleus is small; they are probably derived from lymphocytes. Evidence seems to point to the fact that plasma cells are active in forming antibodies.

Mast cells are common in the adult in all loose subcutaneous connective tissue. In the skin they are found mainly near the hair follicles and small blood vessels and between fat cells. Various investigators found them around capillaries, small arterioles and venules. They are present in the adventitia of the larger blood vessels and in the sheaths of peripheral nerves. Small numbers can be found in and around autonomic ganglia. They are large round or ovoid cells with nuclei and coarse cytoplasmic granules. Their origin is not quite clear. Investigations seem to prove that they contain heparin and histamine in their granules. According to Riley (1959) it is now clear that the mast cell granule is a "metabolically active organelle which responds to changes in its environment as an intracellular osmometer, and, acting in this way, is capable of liberating its content." The histamine release may be instigated by water, trauma and chemical histamine liberators. The nature and action of these chemical histamine liberators is still the subject of world-wide research. They may eventually help to give a better understanding of some of the effects of the massage technique discussed in this book.

The ground substance is a non-fibrillar homogenous substance which varies from a fluid-like to a gel-like state. It is one of the two components of non-fibrillar intercellular substances, the other being tissue fluid, which is related to plasma. It contains proteins, crystalloids, metabolites and gases. The most important of the mucopolysaccharides making up the ground substance seems to be hyaluronic acid. This has the property to bind water and may therefore be very important in influencing the viscosity of the ground substance. An enzyme—hyaluronidase—hydrolyzes it and therefore seems to be responsible for increasing the permeability of connective tissue. The enzyme is probably formed by micro-organisms. The consistency of the ground substance influences to a certain extent the fibre formation.

The white or collagenous fibres vary in size and are in reality bundles of extremely fine fibrils. One theory considered that these fibres form directly from the processes of fibroblasts. Later experimental evidence, however, seems to point to the fact that the fibroblasts produce some material which is passed into the ground substance, combines with it, and so initiates fibril formation (Angevine, 1950). The bundles of fibres branch and anastomose and usually follow a wavy course. The fibres are soft and flexible but so slightly elastic as to be practically inextensible. Under both theories the fibroblasts are responsible for the production of collagenous fibres. The amount of collagenous fibres present in connective tissue will therefore be directly proportional to the number of fibroblasts present. The collagenous element will influence the extensibility and elasticity of the tissue and the mobility of other structures of which it forms an integral part.

Reticular fibres are small branching fibres which frequently form a net-like framework or reticulum. Areolar tissue contains comparatively few reticular fibres, but they are very numerous in glandular organs and between muscle fibres. At the present time it is thought that reticular and collagen fibres are essentially of similar origin. Electron microscopy and X-ray diffraction seem to prove that reticular fibres are probably young collagen fibrils. They later develop, increase in size and form collagen (Angevine, 1950).

The yellow or elastic fibres are much less numerous, are single, and branch and anastomose freely. They are elastic,

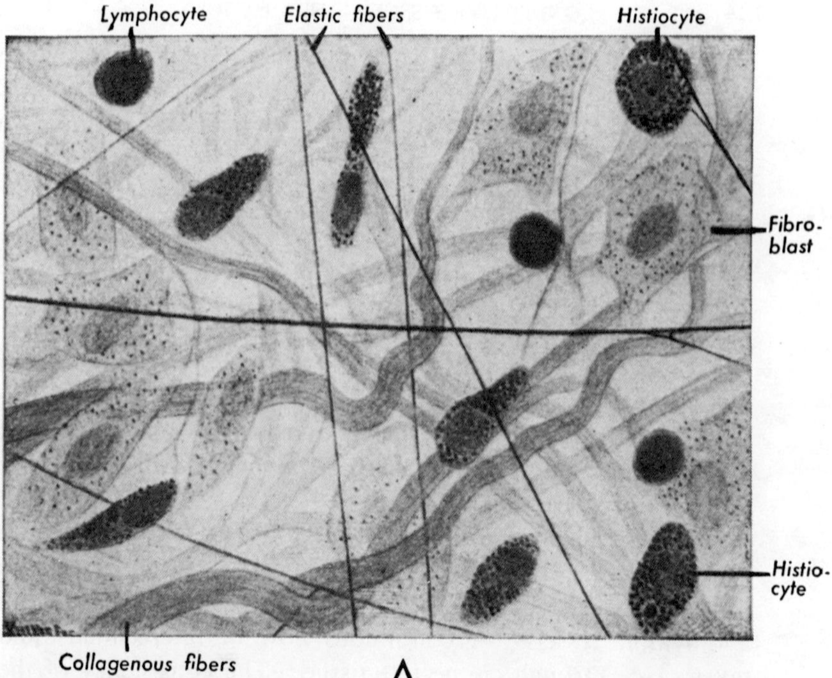
Lymphocyte
Elastic fibers
Histiocyte
Fibro-
blast
Histio-
cyte
Collagenous fibers

A

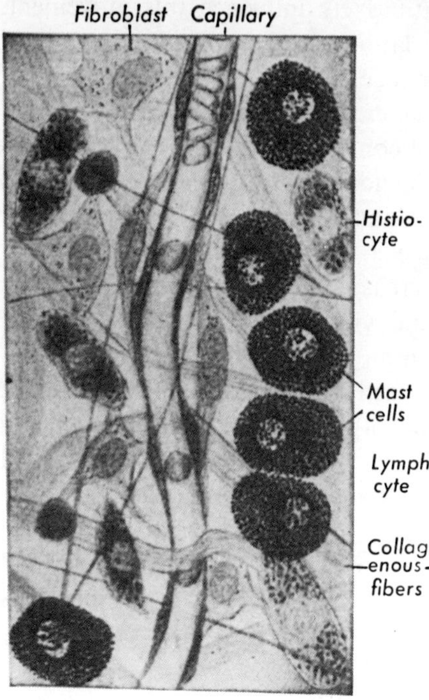
Fibroblast
Capillary
Histio-
cyte
Mast
cells
Collag-
enous
fibers

B

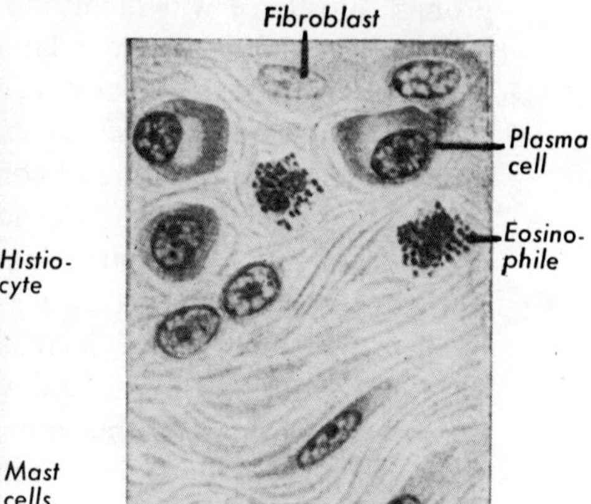
Fibroblast
Plasma
cell
Eosino-
phile
Lympho-
cyte
Fibro-
blasts

C

and are supposed to consist of an albuminoid elastin which reacts differently to various agents as compared with collagen. They are highly resistant to strong acids and alkalis and also resist boiling. Very little is known about the development of elastic fibres. It is assumed that they develop in a similar manner to collagen fibres but at a later stage.

FUNCTIONS OF LOOSE CONNECTIVE TISSUE

Loose connective tissue binds structures together and holds them in position. It allows storage of fat, and so provides a covering which helps to conserve body heat. It plays a significant part in tissue repair by depositing collagenous fibres to form scar tissue.

Nutrient substances pass from blood vessels to the cells of other tissue through connective tissue. In the opposite direction metabolites pass back into the capillaries of blood and lymph vessels. A continuous flow of intercellular fluid takes place through connective tissue. The consistency of the ground substance will quantitatively influence this movement. It will also influence the relationship between fibre material and quantity of ground substance.

It is important to consider briefly some factors which may influence the structure of connective tissue. The hormones of the suprarenal gland and the hormones stimulating suprarenal secretion from the pituitary gland will play an important part. Both fibroblasts and mast cells are influenced by suprarenal cortical hormones. An increase in the hormone decreases the number of fibroblasts and vice versa. A decrease in the hormones will therefore mean an increase in fibroblast activity. Mast cells respond to increased hormones by decreasing in number and size. Lack of hormones will therefore mean increased mast cell activity in relation to hyaluronic acid contents of the ground substance. This will have a water-retaining effect on the tissues. The " Adaptation Theory to Stress " by Selye is interesting in this concept. Thyroxin and oestrogen seem to have similar effects. Iversen (1954) mentions this in relation to the menstrual cycle in women. " Women often become somewhat oedematous immediately before and during the early menstrual period. At this juncture the excretion of oestrogens in the urine increases. They gain weight and the daily output of urine is decreased during these days."

Suprarenal hormones also influence the salt balance of the tissue fluid, this in turn resulting in alteration of osmotic pressure. Retention of sodium and the associated excretion of potassium will result in retention of water and interference with the neuromuscular conducting mechanism. The increased water contents of cutaneous and subcutaneous tissue will affect the capillary circulation of these tissues, and the interference with the neuromuscular conduction mechanism will result in muscular weakness because nervous stimuli are not effectively propagated. Interference with capillary circulation in connective tissue may influence the excretion and synthesis of metabolites resulting from tissue activity.

Clinical experience has proved that the massage technique discussed in this book can effectively increase cutaneous and subcutaneous circulation followed by increase of urinary output. The improved circulation will result in an improved osmotic pressure and H-ion concentration situation.

CHAPTER II

Fascia—Main Fascial Structures in the Extremities and Trunk

THE word " fascia " means " band " and is applied to fibrous or membranous expansions of connective tissue which are wrapped round various structures, especially muscles, and so serve to keep them in definite and intimate relationship. Fascia also forms strong fibrous sheets attached to bony structures dividing the various aspects of the extremities into compartments containing muscle groups of similar function. It is found beneath the skin in almost every part of the body and lodges the final ramifications of vessels and nerves. Under normal conditions it usually permits free movement of the skin on the underlying structures (the soles of the feet and the palms of the hands being exceptions). It shows the typical consistency of connective tissue with a preponderance of the collagenous over the elastic fibre element. Its vascularity will profoundly influence the mobility and function of many structures. Many of the connective tissue massage (C.T.M.) strokes are carried out along fascial structures and attachments. It is for this reason that a summary outline of the significant fascial structures in the extremities and trunk is attempted.

Gluteal fascia

The gluteal fascia is continuous with the fascia of the trunk above and the fascia of the leg below. Above it is attached along the iliac crest, and below it blends with the fascia lata; behind it is attached along the lateral border of the sacrum and coccyx. It sends numerous septa into the structure of gluteus maximus, and it forms a septum between gluteus medius and minimus. Laterally it attaches to the great trochanter of the femur.

Fascia lata

This is the continuation of the abdominal fascia and the gluteal fascia. It forms two septa which attach in the lower femoral region to the shaft of the femur, so forming two definite compartments which divide the flexor group (hamstrings) from the extensor group (quadriceps). In the upper part of the femoral region numerous connective tissue septa are formed to divide the anterior from the posterior muscles on the medial side and allow the development of a third group —the adductors. In the upper and medial part of the femoral region fascial laminae and thickenings take part in the formation of the femoral triangle and the ensheathing of the main femoral vessels. From the apex of the triangle connective tissue forms the subsartorial canal, which ends in the adductor hiatus of the medial intermuscular septum to allow the passage of the femoral vessels to the back of the limb into the popliteal fossa. Laterally the femoral fascia is specially thickened and enforced by the fibres of insertion of tensor fascia femoris and part of the insertion of gluteus maximus. This specially enforced fascial band—the iliotibial tract—carries the insertion of these two muscles to the attachment of the band on the lateral surface of the tibia. This not only carries the action of the two muscles over the knee joint, but also serves as a mechanism which allows an increase in tension in the femoral fascia with far reaching effect on the pumping action on the numerous vessels embedded in the fascial stocking enveloping the thigh. Numerous lymph vessels are embedded in the femoral fascia. The density of the collagenous element of the iliotibial tract may lead to contracture and interference with the function of the limb. On the medial side the fascia also splits to ensheath the insertion of sartorius. The caudal part of the fascia attaches to the femoral and tibial condyles, the fibular head and the base of the patella, and becomes continuous with the popliteal fascia. Medially and laterally from the patella the fascia lata blends with the patella retinaculae and anteriorly with the ligamentum patellae.

Popliteal fascia

This represents the posterior continuation of the fascia lata and is particularly strong. In full extension of the knee it becomes tense and serves as a protection for the popliteal vessels which lie comparatively superficially. The numerous anastomosing vessels of the knee joint region are influenced by tension of the popliteal fascia.

Fascia cruris

The fascia of the lower leg can be divided into deep and superficial parts. The superficial fascia covers the muscles of the limb and forms very important intermuscular septa which provide compartments for the functionally different muscle groups. The anterior septum is attached to the anterolateral border of the fibula, and the lateral septum to the posterolateral border of the fibula. This results in an anterior compartment for the extensors and a lateral compartment for the evertors. Posterior to the lateral compartment can be found, the posterior compartment for the flexors. During muscular contraction these septa form channels which can easily be palpated. The deep tibial flexors are divided by a deep fascial septum from the superficial group of gastrocnemius and soleus. The septa forming the anterior, lateral and posterior compartments are a good guide to the vessels supplying the lower leg.

Fascia pedis

The superficial fascia of the leg continues into the dorsum of the foot. In the ankle region special thickenings are formed which serve as muscular retinaculae. A deep layer of dorsal fascia passes over the interossei. The skin in this region is easily movable over the subcutaneous tissue spaces which may serve as storage places for fluid. On the plantar surface the cutaneous and subcutaneous tissue are closely adherent, some fat being stored between the layers. A thick aponeurosis is developed over the muscle layer. The subcutaneous tissue contains a rich network of blood and lymph vessels and is therefore responsive to C.T.M. The tissue spaces are very small and fluid is not easily retained on the plantar surface of the foot. The deep plantar fascia forms longitudinal compartments for the interossei. These compartments do not divide the plantar from the dorsal structures, and vessels pass freely between both aspects.

Axillary fascia

The superficial axillary fascia shows many perforations for the passage of superficial vessels and nerves. Anteriorly it is continuous with the superficial pectoral fascia and posteriorly with the superficial fascia of the back. Above it blends with the coracocleidopectoral fascia and it is continuous with the fascia covering the muscles which help to form the axillary space, *i.e.* serratus anterior, subscapularis and latissimus dorsi. Between the superficial and deep axillary fascia a space is formed which contains the neurovascular bundle of the axilla. This includes the nervous structures of the brachial plexus and the axillary vessels. Great care is therefore necessary when working in this region. The axillary vein in particular is closely enveloped with connective tissue which attaches it to the clavicle and makes it participate in all movements which open up the axillary space, which is partly filled with loose connective tissue. This tissue also contains the deep and superficial lymph nodes of the axilla which drain the upper extremity, the upper part of the chest wall and the upper part of the back.

Brachial fascia

The superficial fascia of the arm is continuous on the flexor aspect with the axillary fascia and on the extensor aspect with the fascia over deltoid. It envelops the extensor as well as the flexor muscles of the arm and attaches on all the bony prominences. A thickening in the fascia attaches to the lateral and medial supracondylar ridges as well as to the epicondyles of the humerus, thus forming intermuscular septa which divide the arm region into anterior and posterior compartments. Laterally the septum reaches as far as the deltoid tuberosity and medially as far as the insertion of coracobrachialis. The subcutaneous tissue of the upper arm contains the two main superficial drainage veins of the upper extremity, laterally the cephalic vein which passes upwards into the sulcus formed by deltoid and pectoralis major, whence it passes deep to drain into the axillary vein. Medially passes the basilic vein across the medial compartment of the antecubital fossa to approximately the middle of the upper arm to drain into the medial of the two brachial veins. The bicipital fascia which passes medially to blend with the fascia over the common flexor origin, and can be clearly felt as a thickening in the superficial fascia, is a very good guide to the basilic vein. The brachial fascia is continuous with the fascial roof of the antecubital fossa and the connective tissue filling this space, enveloping the neurovascular structures which lie in the medial compartment of the fossa. The superficial lymphatics follow the superficial veins. On the medial side above the medial condyle may be found in the course of the lymphatics a few inconstant lymph nodes.

Forearm fascia

The superficial fascia is continuous with the brachial fascia. It receives strengthening bands from the attachments on the two epicondyles of the humerus and the attachment on the olecranon of the ulna. It is attached for the whole length of the posterior border of the ulna and affords attachment to extensor and flexor muscles, so amplifying the skeletal attachment areas. From the superficial fascia septa pass to the forearm bones to blend with the periosteum. With the help of the interosseous membrane three definite compartments are formed. The first compartment contains the muscles from the common flexor origin and the flexor muscles originating from radius and ulna. It is subdivided by a thin fascial sheet into a deep and a superficial area, dividing flexor profundus, flexor longus pollicis and pronator quadratus from the superficial flexors. The second compartment contains the muscles originating from the lateral supracondylar region of the humerus, *i.e.*, brachioradialis, extensor carpi radialis longus and brevis, and supinator. The third compartment contains the rest of the extensors. Apart from the compartments for the muscles, connective tissue forms definite channels for blood vessels and nerves. The most important channels are the radial channel which can be palpated and contains the radial artery between brachioradialis and the tendon of flexor carpi radialis. The artery gives up at this point the superficial volar artery which passes into the palm of the hand. The ulnar channel, between flexor digitorum sublimis and flexor carpi ulnaris, contains the ulnar artery which also passes into the palm of the hand.

Palmar fascia and aponeurosis

The palmar fascia is continuous with the forearm fascia, having developed thickenings transversely on the posterior and anterior aspects which prevent displacement of the tendons of forearm muscles passing into the hand. The cutaneous, subcutaneous and aponeurotic tissues of the palm of the hand are closely adherent. The palmar aponeurosis is formed by the expansion of palmaris longus and continued into the fascial covering of the muscles of the thenar and hypothenar eminence. Towards the fingers pass star-like expansions which are partly attached to fascial coverings of muscles, but these may pass deep to blend with periarticular structures and periosteum in the region of the metacarpophalangeal joints.

Back

The skin of the back is particularly coarse and thick but becomes thinner towards the mid-axillary line. The subcutaneous tissue is very well developed and loosely woven, so that the cutaneous tissue is easily movable on the subcutaneous tissue under normal conditions. On both sides of the spinous processes longitudinal fibres are found in the subcutaneous tissue which blend with deeper layers. In this area the cutaneous tissue is therefore less movable. This also applies to the lower lumbar and sacral regions where the subcutaneous tissue becomes thinner. The superficial layer of the lumbar-dorsal fascia attaches to the sacrum and the iliac crest. This blends on its deep surface with the origin of sacrospinalis. From it originate the lower fibres of latissimus dorsi. This

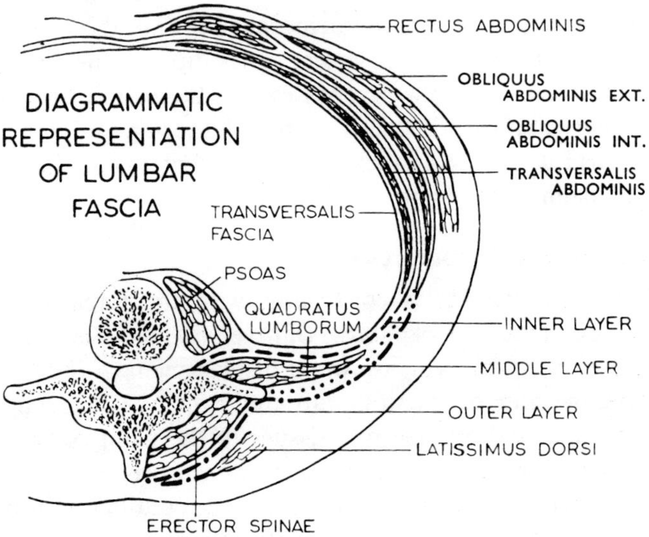

FIG. 2

superficial layer becomes thinner and finally membranous as it ascends cranialwards. The deep layer of the dorso-lumbar fascia stretches between the iliac crest and the last rib. From it originate parts of abdominus obliquus internus and transversalis. Between the lateral border of latissimus dorsi and the posterior border of abdominus obliquus externus a triangular area can be felt with the iliac crest as the base where the abdominus obliquus internus becomes superficial (trigonum lumbale).

Cervical fascia

This can be conveniently divided into three layers.

OUTER LAYER. This is attached above to the external occipital protuberance, the superior curved line, the mastoid process, the styloid process and the border of the mandible as far as the symphysis menti where it unites with the fascia from the other side. It therefore forms a complete hollow cylinder. Below it is attached to the manubrium sterni, the

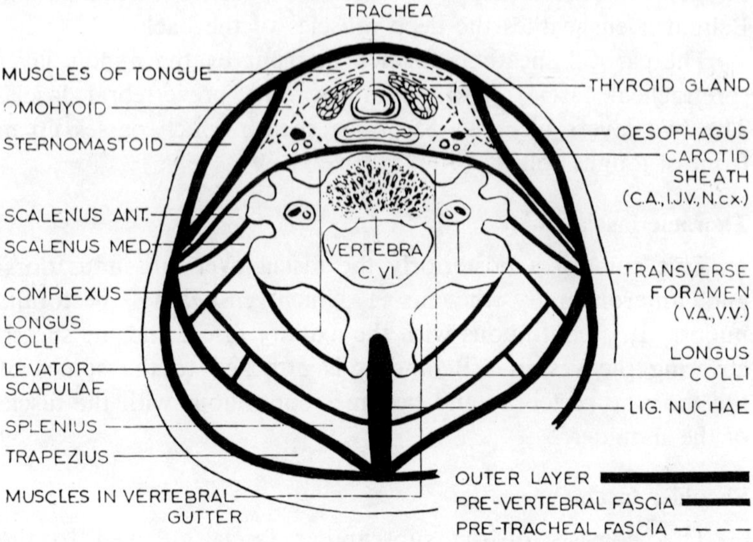

THE THREE LAYERS OF CERVICAL FASCIA

FIG. 3

clavicle, the acromion process and the spine of the scapula from where it blends with the fascia of the back. Behind it blends with the ligamentum nuchae and is attached to the seventh cervical vertebra. It splits twice to form strong sheaths for trapezius and sternomastoid. Any stagnating fluid will therefore be retained superficial to this outer layer, *i.e.* in the subcutaneous spaces.

MIDDLE LAYER. This forms a sheath for the omohyoids of both sides and the muscles of the tongue, and arches between them; it extends vertically from the sternum to the hyoid bone. A prolongation from the sternum forms a sheath for the innominate veins and then continues to blend with the pericardium. It continues also with the sheath round the axillary vessels and nerves.

INNER LAYER (prevertebral fascia). It attaches above to the basilar process of the occipital bone, at the sides to the transverse processes of the cervical vertebrae, and below it merges with the areolar tissue of the posterior mediastinum. Behind it ensheathes the deep muscles of the back.

The carotid sheath is formed in front by the middle layer (pretracheal fascia), and behind by the prevertebral fascia. The two layers blend to form the sheath which passes up in front of longus colli.

Thoracic fascia

This comprises posteriorly the fascia over latissimus dorsi and anterolaterally the fascia which ensheathes pectoralis major. It is continuous with the axillary fascia and the sheath covering the vessels. Behind it is attached to the spines of the thoracic vertebrae and becomes continuous with the fascia of the shoulder.

Shoulder fascia

This consists of the subscapular fascia attached to the margins of the subscapular fossa and covering subscapularis. The supraspinous fascia, which is very strong, is attached to the margins of the supraspinous fossa and covers supraspinatus. The infraspinous fascia is attached to the edges of the infraspinous fossa and covers infraspinatus. This fascia is intimately connected to the fascia covering deltoid. The infraspinous fascia splits to cover deltoid on both aspects, the posterior lamella continuing over the whole surface of the muscle; the anterior lamella blends with the posterior part of the capsule of the shoulder joint.

Intercostal fascia

This consists of an outer layer covering the external intercostal muscles and an inner layer covering the inner surface of the internal intercostal muscles. A very thin fascial membrane separates the two muscle layers. The deep layer is thickened behind to form the posterior intercostal aponeurosis from the tubercle of the rib to its angle; the superficial layer forms the anterior intercostal aponeurosis from the junction of the rib and its cartilage to the sternum.

Abdominal fascia

The most superficial layer is continuous above with the thoracic fascia; below it passes over the inguinal ligament and continues with the superficial fascia of the thigh. It consists of thick areolar tissue which is inclined to store fat. The next layer is the chief fascial layer of the abdominal wall. It blends anteriorly with the linea alba and the aponeurosis of abdominus obliquus externus, above with the thoracic fascia and below with the fascia lata. The deep surface of the abdominal muscles is lined by the transversalis fascia which is attached below to the iliac crest on its inner lip, so dividing the attachments of transversalis and iliacus.

CHAPTER III

The Skin—General Structure

THE skin or integumentum commune envelops the entire surface of the body. Its epithelium is continuous with the epithelium of the external orifices of the digestive, respiratory and urogenital systems. It comprises certain accessory organs which are derivatives of the skin, such as nails, hair and glands of various kinds. It varies naturally in appearance in some regions of the body, being smooth in some and rough and furrowed in others, and adapting itself continuously to external influences which it has to resist in order to protect the body from injury. It varies considerably in thickness. It may be horny and taut in some areas, such as the soles of the feet, and thin and pliable over other areas, such as the medial surface of the thigh. It is nearly waterproof in order to enable a predominantly fluid body to exist in dry air, and can be immersed in fresh water without becoming swollen or in salt water without becoming shrunken. The pigment of the skin protects the body from the adverse effects of excessive ultra-violet radiation. Apart from these protective functions it is one of the most important structures in maintaining the body temperature at a level in which the human cell can live. The varying blood supply influences the amount of heat lost from the body surface and the amount of heat consumed by evaporation of sweat secretion. The sweat secretion makes the skin act as an excretory organ, particularly of water and salts. It participates in the hormone balance of the human body by being able to develop vitamin D when exposed to ultra-violet radiation. The skin contains numerous nerve endings which pick up external stimuli and allow man to adjust himself to his environment.

In every physical examination skin is of the greatest importance. It can be examined easily with the naked eye, and its appearance may reflect pathological conditions not only of organs but also of general disease. Cyanosis of the skin may indicate respiratory dysfunction, while pallor may indicate circulatory dysfunction. There are many alterations in the appearance of the skin which are a most valuable guide to diagnosis for the medical practitioner but would be far beyond the scope of this book.

Skin is normally thicker on the extensor surfaces than on the flexor surfaces, and thicker in the male than in the female. Its mobility depends on the amount of subcutaneous tissue, the amount of adipose tissue and the number of elastic fibres which it contains apart from its thickness. Elasticity and the amount of subcutaneous fat decrease with age and the skin becomes wrinkled. It becomes damaged when stretched beyond its natural extensibility. The skin of the abdomen has the greatest capacity for distension, but the striae gravidarum in women after parturition are signs of permanent tears in some layers of the skin. Similar lines may be found in other parts of the body after extensive swelling or fat loss.

The skin over the whole body is furrowed by a specific pattern of grooves (cleavage lines) which are orientated in such a way as to indicate the direction of elastic tension of the skin.

In the following paragraphs details of skin structure will only be given according to their importance in the application of C.T.M. Appendages of the skin, such as sweat glands, sebaceous glands, hair, hair follicles and nails will therefore not be described.

General structure of the skin

The skin consists of two layers which are completely different in character and origin. The outermost layer is called the epidermis and is derived from the ectoderm; the innermost layer is called the dermis (corium or cutis vera) and is derived from the mesoderm. Below the cutis is the subcutaneous tissue (superficial fascia) which varies from areolar to adipose in character. Irregular bundles of collagen fibres anchor the cutis to the subcutaneous tissue but allow in most parts of the body a considerable amount of movement. The varying thickness of the skin may be due to differences in the thickness of either or both layers. In the interscapular region the dermis is particularly thick; in the palms of the hands and the soles of the feet a thick dermis is overlaid by a particularly thick epidermis. The boundary line between dermis and epidermis is wavy and forms characteristic papillae. The size and number of these papillae vary in different parts of the body; in the palms and soles the papillae are particularly numerous, tall and often branched. In the skin of the abdomen for instance the papillae are low and far less numerous. The arrangement of the papillae usually depends on the mechanical demands in any specific area and the thickness of the epidermis.

Epidermis

This consists of stratified squamous keratinizing epithelium. Several processes are continuously in progress in the epidermis, and on their harmonious integration depends the health of this skin layer. The cells of the deepest layer of the epidermis constantly multiply by cell division; the uppermost layers of these cells are continuously pushed towards the surface; the cells most distant from the dermis undergo a never-ending process of keratinization and the keratin is continuously desquamating from the surface.

The deepest of the epidermal cell layers is the *stratum germinativum*. The cells of the basal layer of the stratum germinativum show short protoplasmic processes which appear to anchor the cells in the underlying connective tissue. The more superficial cell layers of this stratum show protoplasmic processes which form intercellular bridges. They establish intimate contact with neighbouring cells but do not establish protoplasmic continuity. They are often called " prickle cells " and the layer is often called *stratum spinosum*. Active mitosis is taking place in these layers. The next layer towards the surface is the *stratum granulosum*. The name is derived from granules of keratohyalin in the cytoplasm of the cells. The nuclei in this layer already show signs of disintegration. The next layer is the *stratum lucidum.* This consists of several layers of flattened cells where the cell boundaries are no longer distinct. The cytoplasm of the cells is filled with eleidin, the nuclei have degenerated and their places very often appear as vacuoles in the centre of the cell. The most superficial layer is the *stratum corneum.* It is composed of clear, dead, scale-like cells which have a definite horny membrane and are very closely packed. Intercellular bridges no longer exist. The cytoplasm contains the fibrous protein keratin. Soft keratin forms the hornified layers of skin; hard keratin is found in the nails and the cortex of the hairs. The desquamating cells of this layer are continuously lost from the body surface and are replaced from the deeper layers of the epidermis.

Dermis

This varies in thickness in different parts of the body. It consists mainly of connective tissue, but in some areas smooth muscle fibres can be found, while in other areas somatic muscle fibres penetrate the dermis. Smooth muscle fibres occur in considerable number in the skin of the nipple and parts of the perineum. In the face and neck skeletal muscle fibres of the muscles of expression and platysma blend with the dermis. Both smooth and skeletal muscle fibres end in delicate elastic bands which blend with the general elastic network of the dermis. The dermis is arranged in two layers which blend without a distinct demarcation. The more superficial layer is termed the " papillary layer " and the deeper one is known as the " reticular layer." The *papillary layer* is composed of widely separated delicate collagenous and elastic fibres and numerous capillary meshes. The upper surface corresponds in its shape to the under side of the epidermis. The papillary layer is not pierced by the cutaneous appendages but envaginates them. The *reticular layer* is composed of dense, coarse, branching collagenous fibre bundles which form rhomboidal meshes. These fibres are mainly

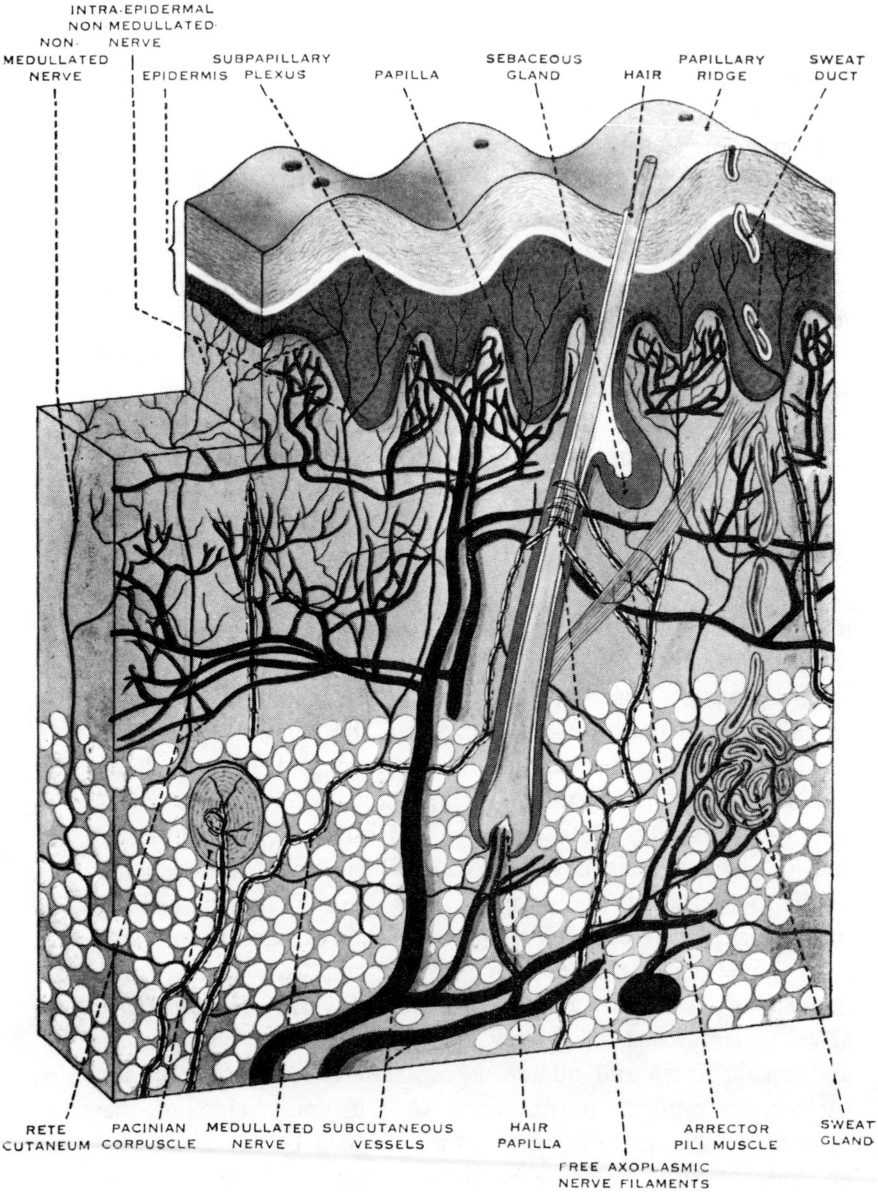

FIG. 4

Diagram of the structure of the skin and underlying tissues; to show the distribution of nerves, arteries, and veins.
(Hamilton, Editor; *Textbook of Human Anatomy*. London: Macmillan.)

arranged parallel to the surface of the skin, and the direction of the main bundles will determine the extensibility of the skin in definite patterns in the various parts of the body. These lines of extension are known as " the cleavage lines of Langer " and are of surgical importance for incisions. Some fibres are arranged perpendicularly and these fibres pass deep into the network of the adipose layer. A network of reticular fibres is interwoven between the meshes of the collagenous fibres. All types of connective tissue cells can be found in the dermal layer. They are more numerous in the papillary than in the reticular region. The most numerous cells are the fibroblasts and mast cells. Under inflammatory conditions histiocytes are present in greater number, which also applies to lymphocytes. Some pigment-bearing and some pigment-producing cells are sparingly distributed in the dermis. The reticular layer contains some ground substance which becomes abundant in oedematous skin. This ground substance exists in a gel-like form in which the water is bound to hyaluronic acid. This bound water passes particularly along the course of the fibres. This layer of skin will definitely be influenced by the manipulations of C.T.M. It might therefore be valuable to consider also the cell element of this layer. The fibroblast is the most abundantly present cell. According to some research workers the fibroblast may be considered the stem cell from which arise all other cells in connective tissue (Montagna, 1956). One of these cells which arise from the fibroblast is the mast cell, which is most numerous in the papillary layer and around capillary beds. A number of conditions show an increase in mast cells (*e.g.*, scleroderma). As previously mentioned the mast cells seem to contain heparin and histamine in their granules. Mechanical stimuli, amongst other factors, seem to induce degranulation (Montagna, 1956).

Vascular patterns of the skin

The dermis of the skin shows a rich vascular supply, while the epidermis, being a true epithelium, is avascular. Most of the arterial vessels of the skin are derived from underlying muscular arteries; very few strictly cutaneous arteries exist except in the scalp and the trunk where the skin receives its vascular supply directly from the intercostal arteries. Arteries enter the skin via the subcutaneous tissue where they form a plexus (rete cutaneum) which lies parallel to the surface in the boundary zone between dermis and subcutaneous tissue. From the rete cutaneum branches pass in two directions. In one direction they pass deep, to supply the adipose tissue in the subcutaneous layer and the hair follicles which lie there; in the other direction they pass through the reticular layer of the dermis, supplying on their way the sweat glands and sebaceous glands. In the boundary zone between reticular and papillary layers they form a second network (rete subpapillare). From this subpapillary plexus arise small arterioles which pass towards the epidermis and give rise to capillaries that extend as loops into the papillae. These capillaries supply tissue fluid to the basal layers of cells of the epidermis. The venous blood returning from the papillae passes through several networks. The most superficial lies immediately beneath the bases of the papillae and receives the blood from the capillary loops. Almost immediately beneath this is a second venous plexus; the two are freely communicating and are often referred to as the "subpapillary venous plexus." A third venous plexus lies at the level of the subpapillary arterial plexus, and the deepest lies at the boundary zone between dermis and epidermis. Spalteholz quoted by Lewis (1927) believes that there are no communications between the arterial and venous side of this vascular system except in the papillae. Apart from these capillary communications, however, there seem to be short direct communications between terminal arterioles and venules—the arteriovenous anastomoses. It might be important to consider the structure of these various vessels. The arterioles deep to the subpapillary arterial plexuses show a strong muscular coat; the terminal arterioles may show a slight muscular element in their structure. The capillaries, collecting venules and venules of the subpapillary plexus are simple endothelial tubes (Lewis, 1927).

Lymphatics

These begin in the papillae and drain into a horizontal network of lymph capillaries in the papillary layer of the dermis. These drain into larger vessels in the subcutaneous tissue to pass out with the blood vessels. The vessels in the subcutaneous tissue receive drainage vessels from plexuses which surround the sebaceous glands, the sweat glands and the hair follicles.

Nerves of the skin

The spinal nerves contain elements belonging to four functionally distinct varieties. These are: visceral afferent, visceral efferent, somatic afferent and somatic efferent fibres. The term " visceral " includes the vascular system with its smooth muscle component. The vascular innervation will be discussed in Chapter V. A very brief survey of the somatic component of the nerve supply to the skin serving exteroreceptive impulses will be discussed now. The surface of the body can be divided into segmentally spaced regions which are called dermatomes. Each of these regions is supplied by a spinal or cranial nerve, the nerve fibres from adjacent regions often overlapping. The cutaneous nerve trunks penetrate the subcutaneous tissue, branch, and send perpendicular fibres into the dermis and epidermis. The specialized endings of these fibres are activated by changes in the environment registering sensations of touch, temperature or pain. On structural grounds they may be divided into three principal groups: (1) Free terminations; (2) encapsulated nerve endings; (3) nerve endings in hair follicles.

Free nerve endings

These fibres eventually lose both their myelin and neurilemmal sheath. The axis cylinder enters the epidermis, and final endings of these fibres terminate among the epithelial cells. Amongst other locations these nerve endings are to be found in the intermuscular connective tissue. Among the fibres ending in this way in the epidermis are also unmyelinated fibres. It is almost certain that these endings are pain receptors. It appears that they can be stimulated by being stretched, in addition to other painful stimuli such as pinprick, etc.

Encapsulated nerve endings

The corpuscles of Meissner are located in the dermis, especially in the papillae, and record tactile sensations. The end bulbs of Krause allow cold perception, the end organs of Ruffini heat perception. Both are found in the dermis. The pacinian corpuscles are widely distributed in the deeper part of the dermis, especially of the hands and feet. They can also be found in association with tendons, intermuscular septa and periosteum. They record deep pressure and serve a two-fold function: (1) exteroreceptive, registering pressure from external sources; (2) proprioreceptive, registering pressure resulting from joint movement.

Nerve endings in hair follicles

These are delicate tactile organs.

SUMMARY

The previously given information makes it quite clear that the skin can no longer be considered to represent only the outer covering of the human organism i.e. the boundary zone between it and its environment. To summarise, it is an organ of protection and excretion, of heat regulation, it produces with the lymph glands antibodies which help to protect the organism against the noxious influences of the environment. According to Professor Niebauer it sometimes overshoots its defensive reaction and produces a variety of allergic manifestations. It also acts as a sensory organ. All these are known facts. These functions are carried out by structures and cells which cannot be found in other parts of the body. This multiplicity of cutaneous functions should be co-ordinated with the rest of the organism. Which is the principal pathway of information and regulation of cutaneous function? Only two pathways seem to be visible with the Electromicroscope i.e. blood vessels and nerves.

Vascular pathways also stand under nervous control so that it seems that the Nervous System must play a dominant role in the normal and pathological processes carried out by the skin. Functionally we distinguish two systems of nerve fibres present in the skin:

1) The cerebro-spinal sensory system
2) The Autonomic (Vegetative) nervous system

The term "Vegetative" seems preferable as no function in the human body is carried out autonomically, every stimulus causes a reaction which eventually spreads throughout the whole organism. The sensory fibres transmit sensory experiences and the vegetative fibres liberate active agents such as noradrenalin, acetylcholine and histamine and regulate in this way, amongst others, the function of the vessels. According to Professor Niebauer the whole sensory influx is retransmitted across the epidermis towards nerve endings which are to be found below the epidermis.

The superficial sensations are classified as corpuscles of Meissner for touch, corpuscles of Krause for cold, Ruffini for heat and Vater for pressure but according to most medical text-books these specialised nerve endings can only be found in smooth areas of the skin, such as the palms, the soles of the feet, the lips and the mammary glands. The sensations can however be observed in many other areas of the body. There are other sensations to be observed such as pain, tickling and itching. The same type of stimulus may produce any of these sensations in different individuals. The same type of C.T.M. stroke, identical in depth and tension may be felt by different patients as "Pain" by others as "Tickle". Present research (Niebauer) suggests that an answer may be found in the difference in molecular structure of various fibres. The clinical significance of these facts will be discussed in Chapter VII.

It is a universally recognised fact that the epidermis cannot function without vegetative nerve supply. The surgical procedure of Sympathectomy attempts to abolish or at least diminish this supply. My own clinical experience proves that with the use of C.T.M. the function can be greatly improved. According to Professor Niebauer's research it may be assumed that the epidermis is formed by two completely different cellular systems. On the one side the epidermis cells consist of keratin forming cells but in between these cells are starlike cells which he called "Dendrite cells." These cells exist in normal epidermis and their connection with the sub-epidermic nerve fibres is observable by electrono-optic research. The triple response reaction takes place in denervated skin. He classifies them as "Neuro-hormonal cells" and considers them responsible for Local Vasomotor reactions which eventually may help to understand processes which via the skin influence the whole organism. This newest research will provide us with knowledge which hopefully may enable us to provide more help to our patients.

CHAPTER IV

The Circulatory System—Structure and Function

THE circulatory system in the human consists of a blood vascular and a lymph vascular system. The blood vascular system comprises a pumping organ (the heart), a series of efferent vessels (the arteries), minute anastomosing tubules (the capillaries) and a system of afferent vessels which return the blood to the heart. In man the lymph vascular system lacks a pumping organ and only consists of lymph capillaries and a system of larger vessels which ultimately form two large trunks. These return the fluid to the blood vascular system via the large thoracic duct on the left and the smaller right lymphatic duct.

Both fluids constitute the internal environment of the body cells. The blood derives the energy which passes it round the body from the pumping action of the heart and muscles and from pressure differences which it meets along its course. The lymph, as far as it is contained in well-defined vessels, will circulate through the pumping action of muscles and through pressure differences. The tissue fluid leaves the channels and is contained in the intercellular spaces. It establishes intimate contact with the cell, and after having fulfilled its metabolic function returns again to the channels. Differences in filtration—diffusion and osmotic pressure—across a selectively permeable membrane are responsible for this fluid movement.

The structure of the walls which form the various types of vessels will influence their permeability. Other factors may also influence the passage of fluid across the wall in either direction and its composition.

The discussion of circulatory factors will be primarily confined to the small vessels which lie near the body surface as these are the vessels which will be influenced in the first instance by the massage technique. It is, however, impossible to influence the circulation anywhere in the body without eventually achieving general circulatory effects.

Capillaries

The structure of capillaries and its influence on the passage of fluid through the wall is an important factor in the attempt to explain some of the effects of C.T.M.

The capillaries are delicate tubes, variable in size in different parts of the body and in different tissues. The capillaries branch extensively and the branches form networks. The density of these networks vary directly with the metabolic activity of the organ. The number of skin capillaries is greater in certain areas, such as the soles of the feet, the palms of the hands and the gluteal region. The meshes of the network also vary in size. They are smaller in more vascular regions and larger in the less vascular regions, such as the calf. The most superficial network will be found near the junction of the middle and outer third of the cutis (subpapillary network). The branches are derived from a network in the deepest layer of the cutis adjoining the fat (cutaneous arterial network). These vessels originate from arteries in the subcutaneous layer of the skin.

The capillary adjoining the arteriole is called an arterial capillary, and the one nearest a venule a venous capillary; the structure of both is identical. The relationship of capillaries, arterioles and venules can be seen in Fig. 5. The function of the capillary network is related to its structure, which is not uniform in all its branches. Some branches originate as prolongations of terminal arterioles and can be traced throughout the bed until they join other similar channels to form venules. These central channels are structurally different from other capillaries and are called metarterioles (Chambers and Zweifach, 1947). Along the proximal portion of the channel the true capillaries branch off and carry blood away from the channel; along the distal portion true capillaries bring blood back into the channel. The difference in structure in the various types of capillary vessels is probably of great functional significance. The proximal portion of the central channel is encircled with single intermittently arranged muscle cells which gradually

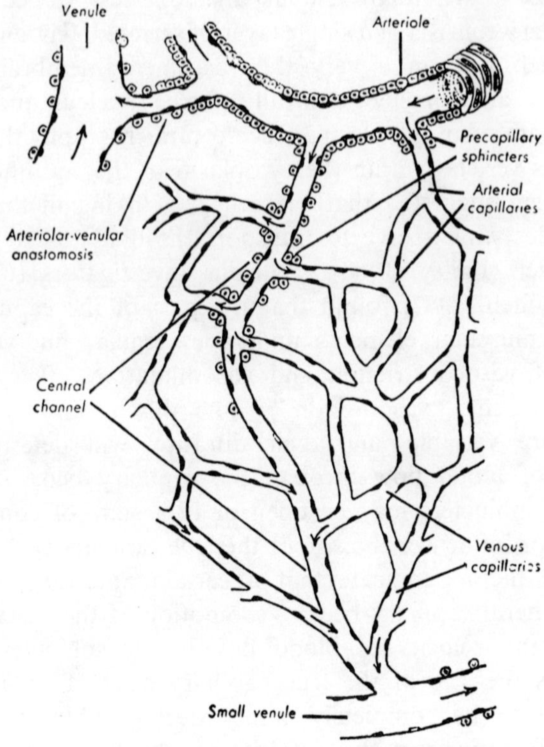

FIG. 5
Relationship of capillaries to arteriole and venule.
(Bailey: *Textbook of Histology*, 14th ed. Baltimore: Williams & Wilkins Co.)

disappear and are completely absent from the distal part of the channel. The junctional segments of the true capillaries are termed "precapillaries." These are also encircled with contractile muscle cells—the precapillary sphincters. Some true capillaries branch off directly from the arteriole, showing also at their beginning precapillary sphincters. These direct offshoots branch into further capillaries which re-unite to join directly with a venule. Some direct shunt vessels passing from arteriole to venule have also been observed. The arterial ends of these vessels show intermittently dispersed muscle cells which are absent from the venular ends. These vessels are termed " arteriolar venular anastomoses." The wall of the capillary consists of a single layer of serrated, flat, endothelial cells which rest on a very thin basement membrane. The cells show an elongated centrally placed nucleus and a clear or finely granular cytoplasm. Electron micrography discovered numerous vesicles within the cytoplasm of the endothelial cell. It has been suggested that the cells, by taking in fluid, form the vesicles which serve to transport the fluid to the opposite cell border (Bailey, 1958). Various investigators (Chambers and Zweifach, 1947) found that the part of the capillary bed showing muscular elements undergoes regular but very slow phases of vasoconstriction and vasodilatation. They termed this movement " vasomotion." The dilator and constrictor phases are variable, and their duration will determine the amount of blood flow through the capillary bed. The precapillary sphincters may be open or in a state of contraction. This factor influences the size of the true capillary bed.

These factors indicate that a certain autonomy exists in the peripheral capillary bed. Vasomotion in the metarterioles controls the velocity of blood flow, while sphincter control influences the size of the true capillary bed. This field does not seem to be completely empty during sphincter closure. Fluid diffuses in from the interstitial spaces and is carried into the distal part of the central channel, returning it to the venules. Resting tissue is comparatively empty. Mechanical, chemical or thermal stimuli decrease vasomotion, the metarterioles and precapillary sphincters open, and hyperaemia results.

Some investigators believe that a specialized cell, the Rouget cell, is representing the contractile element round the capillary wall. Clark and Clark (1943) are in favour of primitive types of smooth muscle cells. The investigation of Chambers and Zweifach seems to indicate that vasomotion is dependent on a nerve supply. The latest experiments of Hilton (1959) open up the possibility of vascular conduction without nerve supply.

The functional significance of the capillary wall lies in the fact that it represents the membrane for filtration, diffusion and osmosis of fluid and filterable substances from the blood stream and back to it. The available surface area is variable and this influences the quantity of the exchange. The movement of fluid and permeable substances is influenced also by the effective pressure on the arterial and venous ends of the capillary field. Effective filtration pressure is normally higher at the arterial end. Fluid therefore passes from the capillary into the tissue spaces. At the venous end osmotic pressure inside the capillary is normally higher and favours reabsorption.

The primary function of capillary circulation is to provide substances for cell metabolism and growth, and to carry away waste products. It also forms an essential part of the body's defence mechanism against injury, such as trauma and invasion by bacteria. The cutaneous capillary circulation plays an additional part in the regulation of body temperature. Alterations in the size of the cutaneous capillary field determine the loss of heat from the body surface. The amount of water loss depends also to a certain extent on the function of the cutaneous capillary field. A small amount of gaseous interchange is also taking place through skin vessels. The important factors controlling the movement of fluid are: (1) the total filtering area available; (2) the properties of the membrane, especially its permeability; (3) the pressure exerted on the fluid inside and outside the membrane. Most of the factors influencing the capillary circulation will act on all three components.

The size of the capillary field is influenced by central and local factors. The central influences affect particularly the parts of the circulation which are known to have a nerve supply derived from the autonomic nervous system. Sympathetic stimulation causes the muscular element of the metarterioles, the central channels, the arteriovenous anastomoses and the precapillary sphincters to contract and so diminish the size of the cutaneous capillary field. This reduces the effective filtering area. Local factors influencing filtration pressure are temperature and position of the extremity. If the extremity is elevated or moderately cool, capillary pressure can be reduced to such an extent that filtration becomes increasingly difficult and absorption is favoured. Trauma, local heat or dependency will elevate capillary pressure, filtration will then be increased and absorption will be diminished. Impedance to the return of exuded fluid will make this fluid stagnant and decrease its oxygen contents. Factors affecting the permeability of the capillary wall are very important, but are still being investigated. Deficiency in calcium or acid *p*H increases the permeability and produces an oedematous condition of the tissues (Zweifach, 1954). Hormonal influences, particularly of the suprarenal and pituitary glands, also seem to affect the permeability.

Arteries

The arteries represent a widely branched network of tubes which carry round the body the blood containing all the substances necessary for cell metabolism. Some run more superficially than others and some are embedded deep in the body tissues. They are tubes which have to resist continuously varying amounts of pressure; the walls therefore live under constant tension. This tension is maintained partly by the inherent elastic properties of the tissue which forms the tubular walls, and partly by variable forces exerted by the contraction of muscular tissue to be found in the walls of most arteries. The muscular tissue is of the smooth variety and its state of tension is influenced by nerve fibres derived from the autonomic nervous system. The nervous control of the muscular element is discussed under Autonomic Nervous System, while this chapter contains only a brief description of the differences of the structure of the walls and their functional significance in the various parts of the vascular tree.

The walls of all arteries are composed of three coats:

(1) the innermost coat or *intima*; (2) the middle coat or *media*; (3) the outer coat or *adventitia*. The structure of these three coats varies according to the size of the artery and its functional part in the vascular system. Three main types of arteries are recognized but the change from one type of artery to the other is a gradual one.

The *large arteries* are often termed "*conducting arteries*." The *intima* of these vessels is formed of endothelial cells and a layer of connective tissue containing collagenous and many elastic fibres which are arranged longitudinally. The deeper portion of the intima contains some longitudinally arranged muscle cells; a few fibroblasts are contained in the more superficial part of the intima. At present there is no evidence that under normal conditions the intima contains any blood capillaries. The fluid environment for the cellular element is imbibed through the endothelial layer from the blood contained in the vessel. The *media* is distinguished by a close meshwork of elastic fibres which is permeated by a very fine network of muscle fibres. The media is by far the thickest of the three coats in these vessels, and there is a large preponderance of elastic over muscular fibres. Both types of fibres are arranged in a spiral fashion. The *adventitia* is a thin coat of connective tissue, mostly consisting of collagenous fibres with very few elastic fibres amongst them. A few smooth muscle fibres are occasionally found in the adventitia. Small blood vessels (vasa vasorum) enter the vascular wall through the adventitia and form a capillary network which penetrates into the media. The large arteries are the aorta and the pulmonary, innominate, common carotid, subclavian, vertebral and common iliac arteries. The structure as described above is most pronounced in the aorta; in the smaller vessels the amount of muscular tissue increases and the elastic tissue diminishes. The main function of the large arteries is to make the blood stream less irregular. The contraction of the heart expels blood at increased pressure into already full vessels. This causes a stretch of the elastic arteries, and part of the force is therefore converted into potential energy. During cardiac diastole this potential energy is converted into kinetic energy, and the recoil of the elastic walls forces the blood along during the rest period of the heart.

The *medium-sized arteries* are also often termed "distributing arteries." They are not all of uniform size and the smaller ones already show a transitional stage towards the arterioles. The walls of these vessels are relatively thick, due to the large amount of muscle fibres in the media.

The intima shows three definite layers: (1) the endothelial layer; (2) the intermediate layer showing elastic and collagenous fibres with a few fibroblasts; and (3) a layer of closely woven elastic fibres. Longitudinal bundles of muscle fibres are often found close to the elastic layer, especially in arteries such as the femoral, popliteal and axillary arteries. The *media* is the largest of the coats. It may show twenty-five to forty layers of circularly arranged muscle fibres, depending on the size of the artery. Between the muscle fibres are networks of elastic, collagenous and reticular fibres. The adventitia blends with the connective tissue of the surrounding area and so attaches the arteries to neighbouring structures. It may contain a few longitudinal muscle fibres. The arrangement of the vasa vasorum occurs in a similar fashion to the large arteries. The medium-sized arteries comprise all the named arteries as far as they are not large arteries, *e.g.*, popliteal, tibial, axillary, humeral, radial, ulnar and intercostal arteries. Due to the thick muscular coat which can contract or relax, the lumen of the vessel can be altered and the main purpose of this type of vessel is to aid in the distribution of blood according to functional demands.

The *true arterioles* still show three distinct coats which gradually disappear as the vessels get smaller and approach the capillary field. All three coats are much thinner; the *intima* consists chiefly of endothelium with very few elastic fibres; the *media* has much fewer layers of muscle fibres; the *adventitia* consists of connective tissue containing all three types of fibres; the *vasa vasorum* are arranged as in the other types of vessels. The outstanding feature in these vessels is that they contain very few elastic fibres, with a preponderance of muscular fibres which are to a great extent under autonomic control. The blood pressure in these vessels has already greatly diminished, and elasticity is therefore no longer important. The main function of these vessels is to control blood flow in the capillary field in the way which has been described under the heading Capillaries. Vasoconstriction or vasodilatation alters the peripheral resistance to blood flow from the larger arteries and is therefore of great importance in influencing blood pressure.

Veins

The veins constitute a system of tubes which serve to return the blood to the heart. The calibre of these vessels as a rule is larger than that of the arteries, but the walls are thinner, due to a reduction of muscular and elastic tissue. Collagenous tissue on the other hand is more abundant than in the arterial vessels of a comparable size. The whole wall is less pressure-resistant and tends to collapse when not filled with blood. A classification into larger, medium-sized and small vessels, as far as structure is concerned, is not possible as the variations in structure do not depend on the size of the vessel but on local mechanical conditions. The muscular fibres are particularly well developed in vessels which are not supported by surrounding structures or are exposed to the influence of gravity in man. A typical example of this type of vessel is the saphenous vein. The resistance to pressure is achieved by a substantial media which consists of longitudinal and circular muscle fibres, supported by elastic fibres. The muscle fibres of venous vessels are probably under nervous control (Ham, 1957). The veins may be divided into two sets, the superficial and the deep, between which are frequent communications. The *superficial* or subcutaneous veins lie between the layers of the superficial fascia and do not accompany an artery. The *deep* veins accompany the arteries, sometimes as a frequently anastomosing pair (venae comites) on either side of the artery, especially in the extremities, *e.g.* radial artery, tibial artery, or as a single trunk running with the larger arteries, *e.g.* axillary artery, femoral artery. In the veins, where return of blood is particularly impeded by the influence of gravity, valves are present to facilitate the return.

VENULES. These collect the blood from the capillaries and have a larger diameter than these vessels and also slightly thicker walls. The walls consist of endothelium which is supported externally by a certain amount of collagenous connective tissue. In the slightly larger vessels of this type smooth muscle fibres may be found intermingled with the collagenous fibres. In the veins of the extremities an increase in diameter of the vessels is usually associated with a more continuous arrangement of muscle fibres. These transitional vessels, from venules to larger-sized veins, are called small veins.

MEDIUM-SIZED VEINS. These include most of the named veins and their branches except the main trunks. They already show the arrangement of three coats. The *intima* is thin and consists of endothelial cells supported by a layer of elastic fibres towards the media. The *media* is the most variable coat in these vessels. It is very substantial in some veins of the extremities, such as the saphenous vein, and very much thinner in the veins of the head. The innermost muscle layer consists chiefly of longitudinal fibres intermingled with elastic fibres, while the outer muscle layers consist chiefly of circular fibres. The *adventitia* is well developed, and consists of collagenous and elastic tissue and often contains a few bundles of longitudinal muscle fibres.

LARGE VEINS. These comprise the large venous trunks of the thoracic and abdominal cavities and the external iliac vessels. The main feature of these vessels is that the media is often very much thinner than the adventitia, in which substantial longitudinal bundles of muscle fibres are developed.

VASA VASORUM OF VEINS. Veins are much more abundantly supplied with vasa vasorum than arteries (Ham, 1957). Veins carry de-oxygenated blood, and the needs of the vessel cells must therefore be supplied from the outside. The vasa vasorum penetrate very often as far as the intima, the pressure inside the vein no longer being a factor to cause collapse of these small vessels.

A special feature of some of the superficial veins is the presence of smooth longitudinal fibres in the intima. Vessels of this kind are the saphenous, basilic and cephalic veins and some of the larger veins such as the femoral and popliteal veins.

VALVES. Veins over 2 mm. in diameter, especially in the extremities, are provided with valves. These are derived from the intima, and consist of loose connective tissue covered by endothelium. A rich network of elastic fibres can be found beneath the endothelium on the surface of the valve directed towards the heart. Most valves show two semilunar flaps which project into the lumen of the vessel and are flattened against the vessel wall when the blood flows towards the heart. Should the blood tend to flow in the reverse direction, the valves float up and occlude the cavity.

Lymphatics of blood vessels

Lymphatics have been found in the adventitia of both arteries and veins. The pressure in venous vessels is very much lower than in arterial vessels. It is therefore much easier for lymph capillaries to remain patent in venous walls. This might explain the greater abundance of these capillaries in the veins.

Lymphatics

Lymphatics represent a collateral system of channels which returns fluid to the blood stream. The fluid contained in free tissue spaces is called "tissue fluid," as soon as it enters a system of channels it is called "lymph." Unlike the blood, lymph circulates in one direction only, from the periphery to the heart. The main function of the lymphatic circulation is to influence not only the quantity of the tissue fluid but also its quality. The endothelium of blood capillaries allows not only crystalloid substances to escape from the blood stream but also a certain amount of colloid substances. It is still generally agreed that escaped colloid substances cannot diffuse back into the capillaries, but they can pass through the endothelium of lymphatics (Ham, 1957). If lymphatics would not return colloids eventually into the blood stream, these would accumulate in the tissue spaces and alter the osmotic pressure, so holding increasing amounts of water in the tissue spaces. It is however realized that the oedema of the tissue spaces is subject to the self-limiting factor of the extensibility of the tissue forming these spaces. The increased hydrostatic pressure of oedematous tissue spaces might cause collapse of lymphatic vessels. The studies of Pullinger and Florey (1935) indicate that the outer wall of lymph capillaries blends with interstitial tissue. If the attaching fibres are stretched by oedema fluid, they tend to pull on the vessels and keep them patent.

LYMPH CAPILLARIES. These vessels start from blind endings in the tissue spaces and anastomose freely to form an extensive network which runs between the blood capillaries. In the skin they are usually more deeply placed than the blood capillaries. They consist of a single layer of endothelial cells, which are exceedingly thin and have a flattened nucleus.

LYMPH VESSELS. The capillaries unite to form larger vessels which resemble the veins in structure. As the vessels grow in size the endothelial wall is first surrounded by collagenous and elastic fibres with a few muscle cells. In the larger vessels three coats can be distinguished: (1) intima, (2) media, and (3) adventitia. In these larger vessels the media consists mainly of circularly arranged muscle fibres with a few longitudinal muscle fibres. The adventitia is the thickest coat and is composed of longitudinal collagenous fibres with interspersed bundles of longitudinal smooth muscle and elastic fibres. The larger vessels contain numerous valves which are arranged in pairs and are constructed on the lines of venous valves. Their arrangement allows flow only in the direction towards the heart.

All the larger vessels empty eventually into two main trunks, the thoracic duct emptying its contents into the venous system at the junction of the left subclavian and left internal jugular vein, and the right lymphatic duct emptying at a similar point on the right side. Hence all the fluid collected by the lymphatic system is returned to the blood vascular system. The lymphatic vessels which lead to the two main draining channels pass on their way through lymph nodes. The reticular meshwork of these nodes serves to purify the lymph and increase its content of lymphocytes.

CHAPTER V

Vascular Innervation

THE heart and blood vessels are innervated by the autonomic part of the nervous system. This is responsible for the control of all vascular and visceral activities. Functionally a clear subdivision into somatic and autonomic components is not possible, as both systems are often closely connected and are interacting. The endocrine system also plays an important part in autonomic activity. The term " autonomic " is therefore used as referring to the part of the nervous system which is directly responsible for the innervation of tissues not under voluntary control.

General arrangement of the autonomic nervous system

The system consists of central and peripheral parts. The central elements are situated in the cerebral cortex, thalamus, hypothalamus, the cerebellum, cerebral peduncles, the medulla and the spinal cord. The peripheral part consists of the sympathetic chain of ganglia, various plexuses and the autonomic fibres contained in most spinal peripheral nerves. The autonomic nervous system is constructed on similar lines to the somatic nervous system. It therefore consists of afferent, intercalary and efferent neurons which are linked as reflex arcs. These reflex arcs, although being essentially automatic are influenced by higher centres. The highest autonomic as well as somatic control is situated in the cerebral cortex. The two parts of the nervous system differ in so far as volitional control of the autonomically innervated structures is in most cases not possible, while the highest somatic control is voluntary.

The autonomic nervous system is subdivided into two parts —sympathetic and parasympathetic. Most visceral structures receive a nerve supply from both parts. The physiological effect on the innervated tissues is antagonistic. It is generally considered that sympathetic efferent fibres are associated with the liberation of adrenaline or noradrenaline, and parasympathetic efferents with the liberation of acetylcholine. Both types of substance are believed to play a part in the mediation of nerve impulses. The exact nature of the effect of these substances is still the subject of intensive research, especially the effect of adrenaline and noradrenaline. Barcroft and Swan (1953) have shown that both substances reduce the blood flow in cutaneous vessels, but adrenaline dilates, while noradrenaline constricts the vessels in striated muscle. Acetylcholine also has differing effects on various arterial structures. It is believed to cause constriction of the coronary vessels but dilatation of other visceral arteries. The terms " adrenergic " and " cholinergic " have therefore been abandoned by some authors and the terms " sympathetic " and " parasympathetic " have been adhered to (Mitchell, 1956). Sympathetic and parasympathetic systems show afferent and efferent pathways.

Sympathetic representation in the spinal cord

It is now universally accepted that the cells in the lateral (intermediolateral) grey column of the spinal cord give origin to sympathetic efferent fibres. They are located in the first thoracic to the second lumbar segments inclusive and are known as the *thoracolumbar* outflow. Mitchell (1953), however, suggested that sympathetic representation is not strictly confined to these regions; it is predominantly found in the thoracolumbar regions because these are opposite areas of maximal visceral supply corresponding to the cervical and lumbar somatic enlargements of the cord where maximum numbers of neurons are required for the supply of the limbs. He suggests that there is sufficient evidence to show that autonomic fibres may enter and leave the central nervous system through any nerves from the first cranial to the last coccygeal nerves, although they are specially numerous in the thoracic and upper lumbar regions. The great majority of sympathetic fibres emerge from the cell bodies contained in the lateral column of the thoracic and lumbar regions as *preganglionic* fibres through the anterior nerve roots. They leave the corresponding spinal nerves almost immediately as *white rami communicantes* to proceed to adjacent ganglia in the sympathetic chain of ganglia. In these ganglionated trunks the fibres may behave in a variety of ways. They may synapse with cells in adjacent ganglia which give rise to postganglionic fibres; they may ascend or descend in the chain and synapse at a higher or lower level; they may pass through the sympathetic chain ganglion without synapsing and continue into one of the prevertebral autonomic ganglia (*e.g.*, coeliac plexus) where they synapse with cells collected in such a ganglion. Each preganglionic sympathetic fibre synapses with a variable number of ganglionic cells. Mitchell (1956) states that there is very good evidence that not all the sympathetic spinal fibres terminate in the way described above. Migrating cells from the neural tube which become arrested during development form intermediate ganglia of varying size which may be situated anywhere along the proximal part of anterior nerve roots or near communicating rami. Some of the fibres emerging from cell bodies in the lateral horn of the cord synapse with cells in these intermediate ganglia. These are very irregularly and inconstantly placed and therefore very often escape in sympathectomies.

The postganglionic sympathetic fibres usually originate in ganglia at some distance from the structures which they innervate, so that their course is usually long and shows a wide distribution. The postganglionic fibres are mainly concerned with vasomotor, sudomotor and pilomotor activities.

Sympathetic postganglionic fibres show a wide variety of pathways. Usually they are very much longer than those from the parasympathetic system. The vessels not very distant from the sympathetic chain receive fibres directly from the nearby trunks. Vessels thus supplied include the aorta and the aortic intercostal arteries, the common carotid, vertebral, subclavian, iliac, lumbar and sacral arteries. The more distant vessels receive their sole or an additional supply through spinal nerves which carry a proportion of sympathetic fibres which enter through the grey rami communicantes. This applies particularly to the more distant vessels in the limbs. Both anterior and posterior primary rami contain sympathetic fibres. Due to the fact that preganglionic fibres of the

DIAGRAMMATIC REPRESENTATION OF CHIEF FUNCTIONAL TYPES OF SOMATIC AND SYMPATHETIC NERVE FIBRES

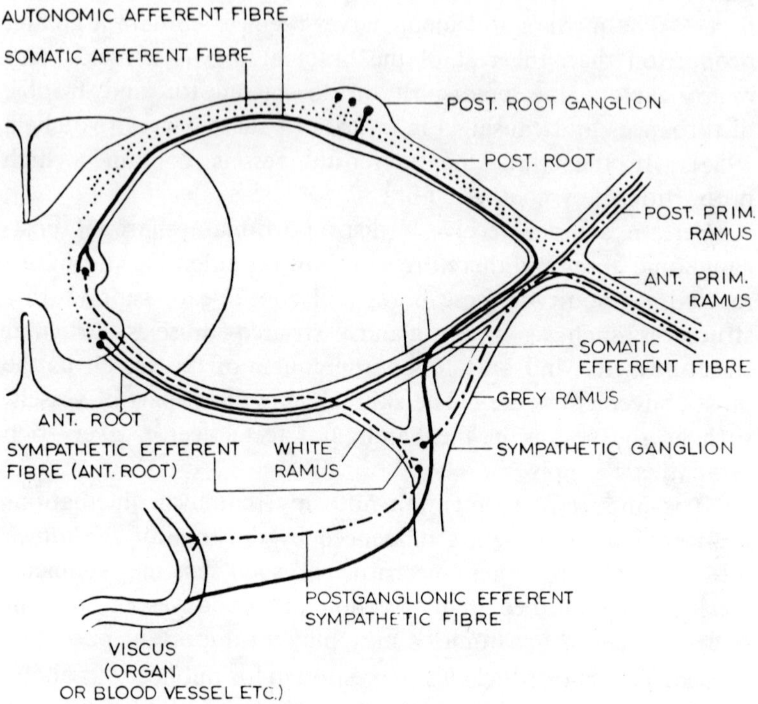

FIG. 6

thoracolumbar outflow may pass upward or downward before they synapse, stimulation of white rami or anterior nerve roots before division produces autonomic responses in several segments, while stimulation of a grey ramus produces responses mainly in the particular segment. The root values of nerves containing somatic and autonomic fibres do not necessarily coincide (Mitchell, 1956). The sympathetic fibres for the lower limbs chiefly emerge through the tenth thoracic to the second lumbar anterior roots, while the somatic efferents emerge from the second lumbar to the third sacral roots. The majority of the vasomotor fibres of the upper limb are derived through grey rami from the stellate ganglion, but may originate from the middle cervical ganglion and receive fibres as far down as the third thoracic ganglion. The nerves of the brachial plexus do not seem to be equally provided with sympathetic fibres. The median and ulnar nerves seem to contain a greater proportion than the rest of the brachial plexus nerves. This might explain the predisposition to vasomotor and trophic disturbances and causalgia in injuries of these nerves (Mitchell, 1956). In the trunk the intercostal vessels contain a high proportion of sympathetic fibres.

Certain arteries receive a disproportionate share of post-ganglionic fibres and therefore will show considerable vasomotor reactivity. Some of these fibres will continue to supply other structures such as sweat glands, striated muscles, articular structures, etc., and only follow the course of the vessels as the most convenient route. The skin and the distal part of vessels, such as the vessels in the hands and feet, receive a very rich sympathetic supply.

It is important to mention not only that local fluctuations in arterial blood flow are influenced by the tone of the tunica media, but that other mechanisms, such as the sphincter mechanism described in the section on blood vessels, present in arteriovenous anastomosis may play an important part.

Since Professor Mitchell's suggestion in his publications about the concept of the sympathetic representation in the spinal cord in 1956 probably is proving incorrect, clinical experience stimulated further research into existing literature on the subject. I was rewarded with a great deal of relevant information. There is now no doubt that the cervical region receives an extensive sympathetic nerve supply. A superficial supply can be found in the cervical region which corresponds to the usual description of the thoraco-lumbar outflow, forming 3 ganglia in the neck. It is however now clear that a second deep supply exists which is derived from the medio-lateral column of the spinal cord at the level of C4-8. (Neuwirth 1960)

Parasympathetic central representation

The parasympathetic preganglionic fibres originate in the nuclei of the third, seventh, ninth, tenth and eleventh cranial nerves and in the grey matter of the middle sacral segments. These are known as *craniosacral* outflow. There seems to be sufficient evidence that preganglionic parasympathetic fibres emerge in the thoracic region via the posterior root and these are known as dorsal root efferents (Mitchell, 1953). These cells may be situated in the intermediate grey matter of the spinal cord. The axons of the cells contained in the cranial nuclei pass to adjacent ganglion cells where they synapse. These cells are contained in ganglia such as the ciliary, otic, sphenopalatine, submandibular, cardiac and pulmonary ganglia. The sacral preganglionic fibres leave the cord in the corresponding anterior nerve roots of spinal nerves as *pelvic splanchnic nerves* and form synapses in neighbouring ganglia. The fibres of the dorsal root efferents are supposed to synapse with cells contained in the dorsal root ganglion or in small ganglia situated on peripheral vascular nerves.

Parasympathetic postganglionic fibres

These arise in the type of ganglion mentioned above and pass directly to the structures which they innervate such as the heart and vessels. This also applies to the pelvic splanchnic nerves. Most of these fibres have vasodilator action. The hypothetical postganglionic vasodilator fibres associated with dorsal root efferents reach their vascular destinations in spinal nerves (Mitchell, 1956).

Autonomic efferent endings

The postganglionic efferent autonomic fibres to vessels pass along the course of these vessels for a considerable distance until they break up to form perivascular plexuses from which small groups of fibres penetrate into the adventitia and media. It is suggested by some investigators (Glaeser, 1928) that a third deep network exists which lies in the zone between the media and intima. Some nerve cells and small ganglia are often found in association with the adventitia of vessels such as the radial artery. These seem to be efferent sympathetic or parasympathetic neurons which have migrated along the vascular nerves. The structure and mode of action of the terminal network round vessels is still very controversial. Explanations of the various theories with extensive reference quotations can be found in *Cardiovascular Innervation* (Mitchell, 1956). Most investigators acknowledge the presence of small cells which are different from connective tissue cells and belong to the autonomic nervous system. They are known as the interstitial cells of Cajal. These cells form a syncytium round the terminal vessels. It is suggested that the postganglionic fibres establish connections with these cells by synapses. Other investigators claim that the postganglionic fibres end in a syncytium. Various theories are brought forward to explain vasodilator and vasoconstrictor effects. No evidence seems to have been found that some of the cells are adrenergic and others cholinergic. Mitchell (1956), quoting Jabonero. suggests that the Cajal cells are capable of reacting in response to different local stimulations. Another suggestion is that two closely interwoven networks exist—one connected with the sympathetic, the other with the parasympathetic nerves.

The most important factor evolving from these investigations is that the existence of a terminal syncytium seems to be established. A spreading response to hormonal or other humoral changes in the environment of the interstitial cell must therefore be expected. This response will be modified if an intact extrinsic nerve supply exists but will be present to a certain extent even if the nerve supply is pathologically (anterior poliomyelitis) or artificially (sympathectomy) absent.

Innervation of veins

The veins as well as the arteries receive a nerve supply on similar lines to those discussed above. The supply seems to be less abundant. The distal vessels in the limbs show a more profuse nerve supply corresponding to a similar arrangement in the terminal arteries.

Innervation of capillaries

The syncytial terminal network is present particularly in the arterial capillaries and round arteriovenous anastomosis: it seems, however, to end at the level of the venous end of the capillary field.

Autonomic afferent pathways

Similar to the somatic afferent system the autonomic afferents are capable of conveying impressions of pain, stretch, pressure and other irritating stimuli by specialized nerve endings to the central part of the autonomic nervous system. The receptor organs consist of free and encapsulated nerve endings which are present in the adventitia or in the immediate perivascular connective tissue especially in connection with vessels of the extremities (Wilde, 1951). Vascular pain sensitivity may persist in areas where other forms of pain perception have been abolished by regional or spinal anaesthesia (Mitchell, 1956). The venous adventitia seems particularly sensitive to painful stimuli.

The origin of these afferent fibres is arranged in a similar pattern to the somatic afferent pathways. The peripheral afferent fibres are the peripheral processes of pseudo-unipolar cells to be found in the posterior root ganglion of the spinal nerves and in the peripheral ganglia associated with the fifth, seventh, ninth and tenth cranial nerves. These afferent fibres may be found in mixed spinal nerves or in purely autonomic nerves. Especially in the limbs, the paravascular afferents accompany the vessels for variable distances before leaving them and joining a spinal nerve through which the impulses are then carried to the cord and brain. This paravascular afferent pathway explains existing pain sensibility along vessels from areas in which the somatic afferent pathways are not functioning. The sensations are transmitted via the cell body of the cell of origin to the central process of the pseudo-unipolar cells and carried either to the spinal cord or to the corresponding centre connecting with the cranial nerve. Similar to somatic afferent impulses they may then take part in the formation of reflex arcs either by connecting directly with a cell in the lateral column of the spinal cord or by means of an intercalary neuron. Some axon collaterals pass vertically and carry impulses to higher autonomic levels. Some axon collaterals may synapse round cells in the posterior grey column and give rise to fibres which eventually may carry these impulses to cortical level.

Summary of function

In the above paragraphs I have attempted to give a very brief summary of some of the structures involved in autonomic function. It is essential to realize that the autonomic nervous system does not work apart from the rest of the nervous system. It is only necessary to mention how loud noise perceived by the exteroceptive system may speed up heart action and so influence the entire circulation. The chronic state of worry and excitement, only too often present in modern times, involving a voluntary part of the nervous system will very often result in pathological conditions involving the autonomic part of the nervous system (*e.g.*, tension headache).

CHAPTER VI

Technique

Principles of application

The autonomic nervous system serves to co-ordinate the various structures of the human body. The structures under autonomic control continue to function as long as the body is alive, and are independent of voluntary control. The severance of a somatic spinal nerve will abolish the function of the organ which it supplies. The severance of an autonomic nerve will not interfere with the function of the supplied organ during the resting state. The heart with all autonomic connections severed will continue to beat, provided its nourishment is maintained. The impulse for its basic function arises in the organ itself. The function of the autonomic nervous system is to co-ordinate the various structures and make them adaptable to varying and changing stimuli arising from changes in the environment. The autonomic centres serve to modify the reaction to peripheral stimuli of somatic and autonomic origin, and establish harmonious interaction of structures under somatic and autonomic control, *e.g.*, thermal stimuli registered by the terminal somatic nerves will cause adaptive constriction or dilatation of peripheral blood vessels. The close interrelation between the somatic, autonomic and endocrine systems makes it impossible for pathological changes to take place in any one structure without causing adaptive changes in other structures.

Surface changes relating to sensibility and contour in organic pathological disturbances have already been reported by Head in 1898.

Capillary changes in skin segments within the dermatome supply of a pathologically affected organ have been investigated microscopically by Dittmar (1943) and by Rouanet (1946).

Changes in muscular tension and pain sensibility have been

discussed by Mackenzie (1917) and others. The most universally known example is the circumscribed abdominal tension in appendicitis.

The pathway responsible for peripheral changes in pathological organic disturbances may also be responsible for changes in the opposite direction. Hartmann (1928) describes changes in connective tissue within the dermatomes of the heart, causing heart symptoms and clearing up after treatment of the peripheral connective tissue.

Nonnenbruch and Gross (1952) describe similar phenomena which they investigated. These observations should prove that body surface, organs and connective tissue within the segmental nerve supply are connected by reflex pathways. Changes in one part of the segment may be responsible for alterations in other parts of the segmental supply. The previously described distribution of autonomic cell stations and fibres will have made it clear that tissue changes due to alteration in blood supply will not remain confined to one particular segment. Treatment of peripheral changes should therefore be continued until the circulation over the whole body surface is normalized to the greatest possible extent. Hypersensitive zones must disappear before terminating the treatment.

Pathways concerned may be as follows, choosing stomach pathology as an example: The stomach is supplied by the great splanchnic nerve which derives its fibres from the segments T.5 to 9. Ascending sympathetic branches pass to cervical ganglia from the same segments. Maximal points for stomach pathology lie in the dermatomes of C.3 to 4 and T.5 to 9.

VISCERO-CUTANEOUS. Afferent from stomach—Posterior Root Ganglion (P.R.G.)—lateral horn cell white ramus—sympathetic ganglion—grey ramus—somatic nerve carrying fibres to blood vessels.

Result. Vasoconstriction in the periphery and hyperaesthesia. Changes in subcutaneous tissue.

CUTANEO-VISCERAL. Altered tension in the periphery registered by posterior afferent—P.R.G.—lateral horn—sympathetic ganglion—postganglionic fibre to stomach.

Result. Interference with stomach blood supply and new flare-up. The peripheral changes are invariably present but usually clear up within two to three weeks. For unknown reasons they sometimes do not clear up and cause new flare-up.

VISCERO-MOTOR. This is a variation of the viscero-cutaneous effect, except that the connector fibre establishes a relay into the anterior horn. The new fibre carries excitatory impulses to muscles within the segmental supply.

Result. Alteration in muscle tension.

Investigation before treatment

The present tendency in all branches of Medicine - diagnostic as well as therapeutic - is towards specialisation. In many cases this is detrimental to the final recovery as it leads to a symptomatic approach both in Diagnosis as well as in Therapy. Too much emphasis is placed on the use of machines for Diagnosis as well as Therapy. Art is changing into technique. We have been blessed with the functions of the brain, of organs like the eyes and ears and peripherally placed sense organs in the hands which report back to the brain the state of the environment in which we live and to which we react. We must therefore learn again to see and observe the patient as a whole (global or wholistic approach), obtain his or her account of pain and inadequate function and learn to interpret these factors both in diagnosis and in therapy. We also must consider that every therapeutic measure affects the whole patient. This does not only apply to Drug-therapy but also to Physical therapy.

Although patients are usually aware of alterations in function of joints, muscles, nerves and organs, they are not aware of alterations in connective tissue tension and mobility. While it is obviously important to establish the degree of malfunction in all structures and detect the areas of pain, it is essential to look for the reason of the disturbed function. Very often we fail to recognise where the lesion started, what caused it originally and what changes took place before the disability forced the patient to seek help. The most important factor is to find out if the lesion is of organic origin, or due to faulty use or trauma affecting the mobility apparatus during work or leisure, if scar tissue of various kinds interferes with certain structures. It is also to be considered if changes in the tension of surface tissues are due to the presence of stress situations which the patient could not manage. The changes in connective tissue unobserved by the patient can be detected by the therapist to a great extent by inspecting the back. The result of the *Back Inspection* and the information gained from the patient during the procedure will make it possible to make an informed, reasoned approach to the treatment and thus help to shorten the treatment period and make it more effective. This approach does obviously not exclude investigations such as X-ray etc.

Back Inspection

The aim of the Back Inspection is therefore to find out if *visible* changes can be detected in the surface contour of the back which may be due to tension alterations. These changes may be caused by inflammatory processes which have taken place or are still taking place in an organ which shares the same embryological nerve supply with surface tissues in certain well defined areas. The inflammatory condition in a viscus will draw a greater fluid supply to that organ and therefore deprive other tissues within the segment of their fluid supply and cause alterations in their consistency. The surface tissues in the associated area will therefore appear drawn in and can be detected as flattened areas (Head's zones). As the vegetative vascular pathways are widely interrelated changes and irritations must also be expected in more distantly situated areas. This is important for treatment and diagnosis. The degree of changes and irritation in various segments will differ. The most affected zones (maximal points) will often be a guide to the origin of the lesion. As connective tissue is also part of muscle structure, the disability may extend into impaired muscle function. The tension changes will not only affect the mobility of surface tissue layers but also their sensibility. (Ebner 1978)

Technique of investigation

The patient is in the sitting position where this is possible. It may be advisable to carry out the *treatment* in the forward lying, or side lying position, especially in circulatory conditions. The initial investigation will be more reliable if carried out in the following position: sitting, back straight, pelvis slightly tilted forward to shorten the back muscles and make cutaneous tissue movable. Hips and knees at right angles. Feet fully supported. Hands resting on the thighs. The slight postural contraction necessary to maintain this position allows movement of the skin on the subcutaneous tissue. This is the position of choice for treatment, except when treating the lower extremity. If the patient's condition makes it necessary, both investigation and treatment positions must be adapted accordingly. Side lying as a position has the disadvantage that the two sides of the body cannot be compared.

The nerve roots of arm and leg segments originate from the back. This explains the importance of the back for investigation and for treatment.

Visible investigation

This is carried out to find alterations in the contour of the back. Tension in subcutaneous tissue can be more easily recognized in the buttock areas, the sacral area, between the scapulae, and over the scapulae. Changes in the thoracic region are less reliable. In most adults the paravertebral areas are not strictly symmetrical. Right or left handedness, especially in manual labourers, influences the contour of the back; the habitual sitting position of desk workers causes permanent changes in the tension of the postural muscles. These small habitual postural deviations which cause no disability to the patient will influence the back contour without being of importance. All these lesser changes are easily recognized by the experienced worker.

Importance of observed changes

Changes in the lower sections of the back, the sacral region and the shoulder region, are always significant. Changes in the thoracic region are less reliable. Drawn-in zones are more important than zones of elevation.

Visible reflex zones in subcutaneous and cutaneous connective tissue

Organs receive their autonomic nerve supply primarily from the homolateral part of the nervous system. Connective tissue changes can therefore be found on the corresponding part of the body surface. Liver, gall-bladder, duodenum, ileum, appendix, ascending colon and hepatic flexure receive their nerve supply mainly from the right. Heart, stomach, pancreas, spleen, jejunum, transverse and descending colon, sigmoid colon and rectum receive their nerve supply mainly from the left.

Changes relating to the bladder, the uterus and the head can be found in the middle of the back. Changes relating to the lungs, bronchi, kidneys, suprarenal glands and ovaries can be found on the corresponding side of the back. Conditions affecting the nerves or vessels on either side of the body will cause changes on the corresponding side of the back.

The changes which can be observed visually may be grouped under the following headings:

Drawn-in bands of tissue.
Flattened drawn-in areas of tissue.
Elevated areas giving the impression of localized swelling.
Atrophy of muscles.
Hypertrophy of muscles.
Bony deformities, especially of the spinal column.
Shortening of muscles (*e.g.* latissimus dorsi).

The changes described below follow on the whole those described by Teirich-Leube (1960) which are confirmed by the author from personal experience.

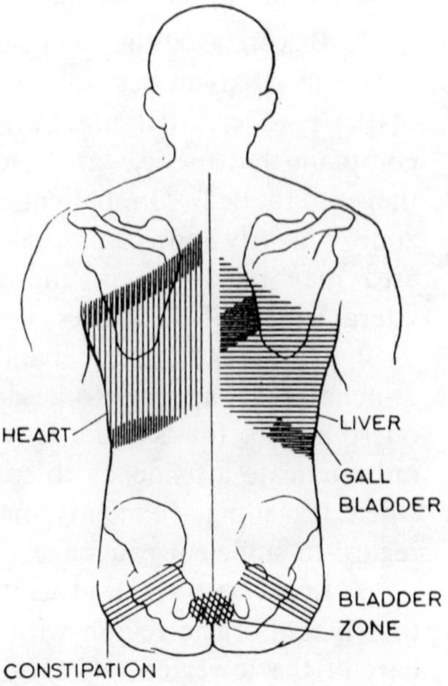

FIG. 7
Visible connective tissue zones 1.

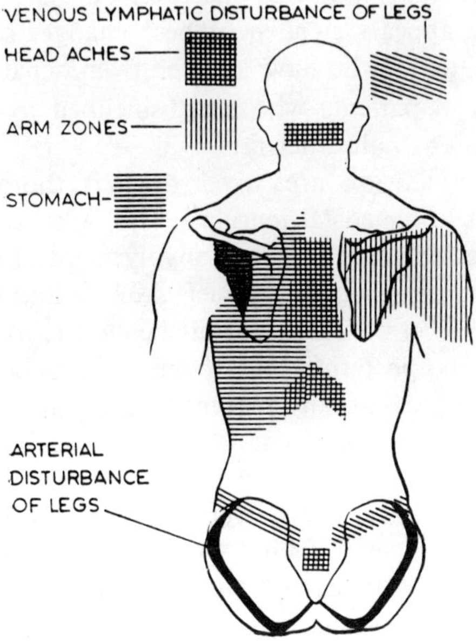

FIG. 8
Visible connective tissue zones 2.

Visible zones in the subcutaneous connective tissue of the back

1. Bladder zone. Half-crown area above the anal cleft drawn in. Patient has suffered or is suffering from disturbances of the bladder. Patients may suffer from cold feet and often complain that the legs are cold up to the knee, especially when they go to bed. In patients suffering from rheumatism this zone is nearly always present; additionally the iliotibial tract area may be drawn in and swelling may be present on the lateral aspect of the ankles.

2. Constipation. A band of tissue, approximately 2 to 3 inches wide, appears to be drawn in, passing from the middle one-third of the sacrum downwards and laterally. It may only indicate a tendency to constipation such as patients suffer when travelling. Patients may have to watch the diet with regard to sufficient roughage.

3. Liver and gall-bladder. A large drawn-in area over the right thoracic region with a special band along the lateral part of the lower costal margin. A smaller area can often be found passing from the lower part of the vertebral border of the scapula to the vertebral column at the level of T.5 to 6. The area over C.7 often appears swollen. These changes may be present not only in patients who have suffered from hepatitis or gall-stones, but also in patients who are disinclined to eat fatty foods or prefer butter to all other fats.

4. Heart. Increased tension area over the left thoracic region including the left lower costal margin. The right costal margin may also be affected slightly, due to involvement of the hepatic circulation. The area between the left scapula and the vertebral column at the level of T.2 to 3 and below the axilla is specially drawn in. The posterior wall of the axilla appears thickened. These changes are usually present in coronary and valvular diseases of the heart.

5. Stomach. Largely overlapping tension areas with heart zones. A typical tension area can however often be observed below the lateral part of the left scapular spine. This area is almost invariably present in all cases of gastritis and gastric ulcers.

6. ARTERIAL DISEASE OF LEGS. The buttock area is changed in sitting; from being square it becomes V-shaped. This is always present in all circulatory disturbances accompanied by angiospasm. The shape of the buttock is a good guide to the severity of the condition.

7. VENOUS LYMPHATIC DISTURBANCE OF THE LEGS. A drawn-in band can be observed passing from the middle one-third of the sacrum, parallel to the iliac crest laterally and forward over the gluteus medius. The patient reports that the legs easily swell up in the summer, on a journey or when staying in a hot room. The patient may suffer from cramp in the calf, varicose veins and/or paraesthesia, especially in the foot or on the outer side of the calf. If the tendency is present in both legs, the zones are present on both sides; otherwise they are present only on the affected side. The severity of the drawn-in area indicates the more severely affected side.

8. HEAD ZONES. Characteristic is the drawn-in area in the thoracic region between the scapulae. This zone seems to be present in all types of headache independent of the cause. It may be present in chronic headache without apparent cause, in migraine, rheumatism, arteriosclerosis, insomnia, often after concussion, osteoarthritis of the cervical spine, disc lesion, etc.

9. ARM ZONES. Drawn-in areas are present over the scapula extending over the posterior part of deltoid. These areas are always present in patients suffering from circulatory disturbances in the hand, nocturnal paraesthesia, neuritis or neuralgia.

Manual investigation

The purpose of this investigation is to obtain a picture of the mobility of the different layers of connective tissue on the body surface and their consistency. Information can also be obtained if any of these tissues are painful on palpation or lack sensation. Palpation of muscles will give information as to the degree of tension present, the uniformity of tension on both sides of the vertebral column or any asymmetry or muscle imbalance, and the presence of small areas of increased tension, especially in muscles such as the upper fibres of trapezius, the

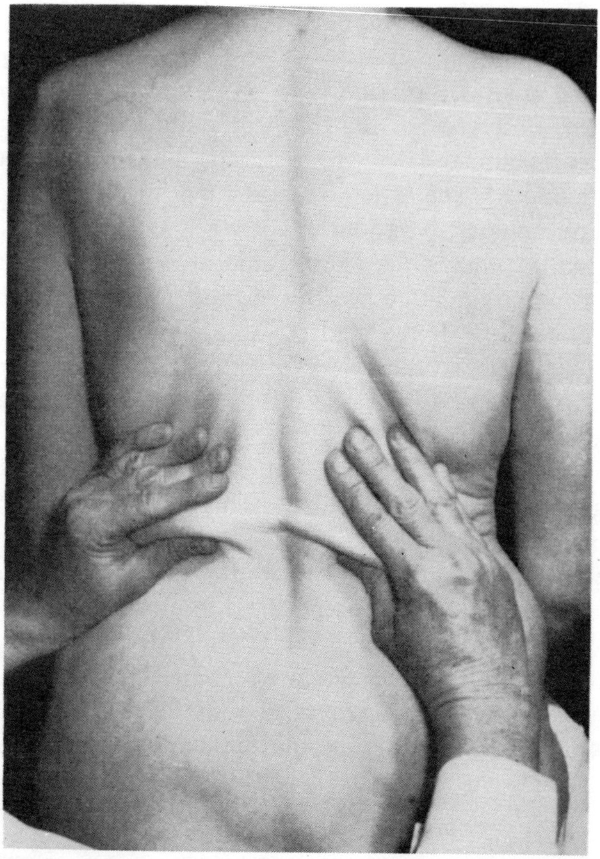

FIG. 9

Manual investigation.

Lifting of skin folds.

extensors of the cervical spine, latissimus dorsi and sternomastoid. The techniques used are as follows:

1. Lifting of skin folds in the direction of the original cleavage lines. The skin is gripped between thumb and fingers, great care being taken not to pinch the skin fold. The fold must be deep enough to allow a lifting away from the fascial layer. This technique is carried out beginning at the lower costal margin and progressing upwards as far as the shoulder region. In some areas it may be impossible to lift the folds from the underlying tissue. On the right this may not be possible in liver and gall-bladder affections or on the left in heart and stomach conditions. Over the scapular areas this immobility may exist in circulatory disturbances of the arms.

2. Technique to test mobility of small areas of superficial on deeper tissues. The slightly flexed fingers of both hands are placed on the body surface, only using sufficient pressure to obtain adherence between the finger-tips and the patient's skin surface. The following areas are investigated:

(*a*) From the buttocks towards the lateral border of the sacrum to obtain information about existing arterial or constipation zones.

(*b*) From the area behind the great trochanter of the femur towards the sacro-iliac joints to obtain information about existing venous lymphatic zones.

(*c*) From the area above the great trochanter towards the iliac crest to obtain information about existing venous lymphatic or arterial disturbance of the legs.

(*d*) Over the sacrum, working from the apex towards the upper sacral segments to obtain information about existing bladder or headache zones.

(*e*) Over the lumbar region on either side of the vertebral column, again working from inferior to superior areas to obtain information about kidney zones.

(*f*) On either side of the vertebral column over the lower costal areas following the direction of the ribs. To obtain information on the right about liver and gall-bladder zones, on the left about heart and stomach zones, and on both sides about pulmonary zones.

(*g*) Following the same direction between the scapulae for headache zones.

(*h*) Over the scapulae from the inferior angle towards the spine of the scapula to obtain information about existing arm zones.

TESTING OF TISSUE MOBILITY

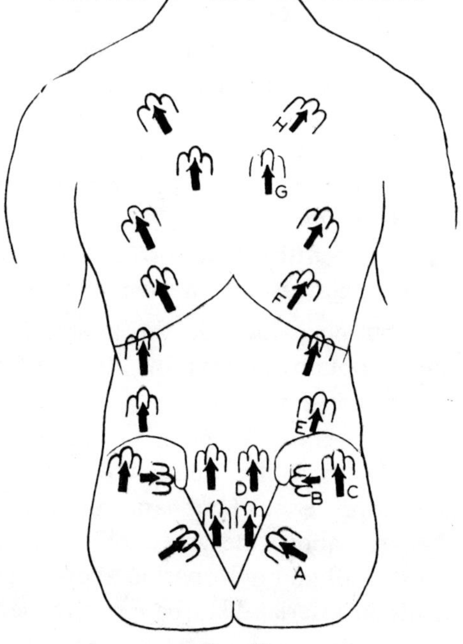

FIG. 10

3. A stroking technique which gives information about the circulatory response of the tissues under investigation. A stroke is performed on either side of the vertebral column, using the third finger supported by the fourth finger at an angle of approximately 40 to 60 degrees. It is essential that all strokes are performed in such a way that tension results on the tissues ; they must not be pushed in front of the investigating

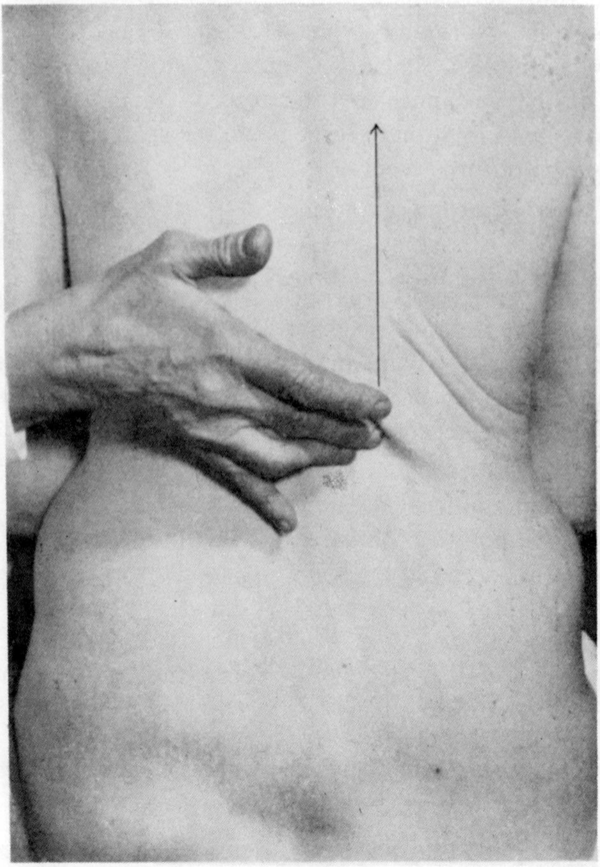

FIG. 11
Manual investigation.
Stroking technique along the vertebral column.

fingers, therefore the wrist of the performing hand must always lead. The diagnostic stroke must not be carried over the sacrum as this may lead to uncomfortable sensations for the patient. Normally a fluent fold passes in front of the investigating fingers; in cases of great tension the finger may become arrested and must not be forced through the tissues. The patient's sensation in response to the stroking investigation may be one of three types:

(*a*) A cutting sensation } both of varying intensity.
(*b*) A scratching sensation }
(*c*) A feeling of dull pressure.

In interpreting the changes found at the manual investigation it is necessary to take into account normal differences of tension which exist in patients of varying types and ages. The main normal differences to be taken into account are:

CONSTITUTION. In a fat person with a great deal of subcutaneous adipose tissue, tension will naturally be greater all over the body as compared with a thin person.

AGE. An old person's skin will normally feel looser all over the body as compared with a young person.

ANATOMICALLY TIGHTER ADHERENCE. In some areas, *e.g.* over the lumbar region, the skin is normally less mobile than over the thoracic area.

Interpretation of changes found by different techniques of investigation

The purpose of the investigations is to discover variations in tension in the subcutaneous and cutaneous tissue and changes in mobility. It is, however, incorrect and misleading to assume that in all cases where such changes are found an organic disturbance exists or has existed. Three possibilities might first of all be considered.

1. The patient has been referred with a diagnosis of definite pathology and the changes found correspond with the expected picture. As treatment with C.T.M. progresses, the symptoms and changes in the superficial tissues improve. Sometimes

both disappear simultaneously and the patient is discharged symptom-free. Sometimes the symptoms disappear completely, and the changes found at the first investigation improve considerably but slight alterations can still be detected. The author's experience and the experience of German workers indicate that these patients very rarely return with the original symptoms.

2. Some patients are referred with a definite diagnosis and the picture on investigation is as expected. Under treatment these patients improve fairly quickly, their symptoms gradually disappear completely and their general health and feeling of well-being show great improvement. The alterations in connective tissue found on investigation do not however improve to the same extent. In these patients freedom from symptoms may be obtained lasting for long periods, sometimes several years, but it may be necessary to resume treatment after an interval of time.

3. Some patients are referred for certain pathological disturbances and on investigation it is possible to find not only the expected alterations but additional zones. On careful investigation it may be possible to find that earlier in life the indicated disturbances existed but at the present moment no corresponding disabilities are reported by the patient. It may also be found that a certain liability to disturbances exists which only becomes apparent under conditions of stress. A patient may, for instance, be referred for treatment because of circulatory disturbances in the arms. On investigation a distinct headache zone is found between the scapulae. During a careful discussion the patient mentions that periods of heavy fatigue bring on fairly severe headaches, while normally he does not suffer from headaches. Another patient without a headache zone may become heavily fatigued without ever suffering from headaches.

According to Teirich-Leube (1960) zones which have never given rise to any symptoms may exist in otherwise healthy people. These zones indicate a certain constitutional type in the same way as we consider certain constitutional types of body build. They indicate that a certain liability exists for these organs to be affected if autonomic disturbances arise as a result of stress reaction. (The term " stress diseases " is frequently used now in the literature, especially in connection with rheumatic diseases where it is realized that the stress factor is very important). The Germans call these zones " silent zones." They are interesting because they may indicate where symptoms may arise under conditions of stress.

It must be emphasized that any discussion with the patient must be conducted very carefully. Questions asked must never be suggestive to the patient. Neglect of this precaution may result in the production of symptoms on the patient's part, or the patient may report to the doctor that the physiotherapist has diagnosed some particular disease. Such a situation would only lead to a disturbance of the relationship between doctor and physiotherapist. The physiotherapist's job is to treat the patient—not to diagnose his disease. It may, however, be important to discuss the situation with the doctor.

Response to diagnostic stroke

The patient may report a feeling of dull pressure in some areas instead of the scratching or cutting sensation. These areas are usually situated in the upper parts of the back, and indicate that areas of deep congestion exist, while areas of more superficial tension still exist more caudally. The intensity of the scratching or cutting sensation in response to the stroking finger is a fairly reliable guide to the amount of tension present.

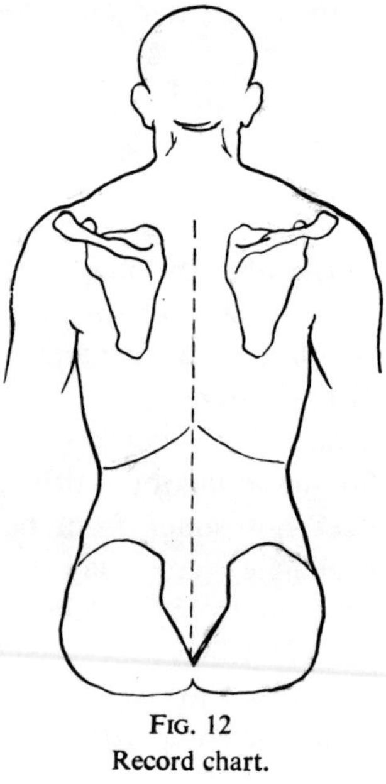

Fig. 12
Record chart.

Records

Before the first treatment it is essential to investigate every patient very carefully and note down the findings. These investigations should be carried out with an absolutely open mind and not with the intention of finding certain alterations.

Duplicated diagrams of record charts will save time when noting the changes found at the first investigation.

General considerations relating to massage technique

It is essential to obtain a clear picture of existing tension areas in order to be successful in the application of the massage. During the early treatment sessions areas of pathological tension and treatment areas may not coincide. The patient must be taught that treatment areas and areas which cause discomfort and show pathological symptoms may not be identical, *e.g.*, paraesthesia of the hands often disappears when sacral and lumbar sections of the back, including the subcostal area, are treated. During later treatment sessions it will be necessary to include all areas which show abnormal tension. Assuming that the caudal areas show abnormal tension or that the circulatory response is unsatisfactory it is inadvisable to progress cranialwards. Eventually however, it will be necessary to include all areas in the treatment in order to obtain lasting results. The chapter on cardiovascular innervation explains how viscera, blood vessels, nerves, muscles and connective tissue are interdependent in their innervation. It follows a pattern not fully understood. The work of Travell (1951) gives an account of how myofascial trigger areas do not follow simple segmental distribution. In all cases, including some of the peripheral circulatory disturbances, the massage should start in the sacral area of the back. This makes it possible to find out if a circulatory pathway between central and peripheral areas can be established. In many conditions this will be the case. In some conditions, however, central stimulation will not produce fully satisfactory peripheral reactions. In the author's own experience this is sometimes the case in poliomyelitis. It seems that the connections between central cell stations and peripheral reticulum are disturbed. In these exceptional cases it is advisable to treat the peripheral areas first. During peripheral treatment of such cases the patient often suddenly experiences a slight irritation in the back which becomes apparent to the operator by involuntary slight scratching attempts on the patient's part. At that point return to the central areas will result in satisfactory peripheral circulatory reaction. Another point related to the arrangement of autonomic cell stations deserves care in the arrangement of early treatment sessions. The stimulation of areas close to the vertebral column may produce undesirable visceral reactions, such as sudden dyspnoea or palpitations. These areas receive their vascular innervation to a great extent from fibres close to the sympathetic chain. As explained under vascular innervation, the preganglionic fibres pass from the lateral horn of the spinal cord into sympathetic ganglia, where they may arborize round a number of ganglionic cells. These fibres may also pass up or down the chain of ganglia to arborize round distally situated cells. It is therefore far more difficult, while stimulating these paravertebral areas, to confine the effect to the treatment area. A very widespread reaction may often result. It will be safer, in all cases where this reaction is distressing for the patient, to treat the lateral areas of the back first. This applies particularly to the lumbar and thoracic segments. The vascular structures in these lateral areas are supplied to a great extent by postganglionic fibres arising in the treatment areas, and effects are therefore much more localized, *e.g.*, should treatment of the thoracic section produce undesirable effects, the stimulation of the latissimus dorsi border will open up peripheral vascular channels and discomfort to the patient can be avoided. Many of the lumbar preganglionic fibres descend into the sacral region; a number of these fibres ascend. This interrelation of all autonomically supplied structures makes it advisable to start every treatment in the sacral area to make certain of a normal vascular reaction at the root of the autonomic supply tree. It is however important to progress as soon as possible into the affected segments. The final aim of all C.T.M. treatment is to normalize, within the limit of still functioning vascular pathways, the tension over

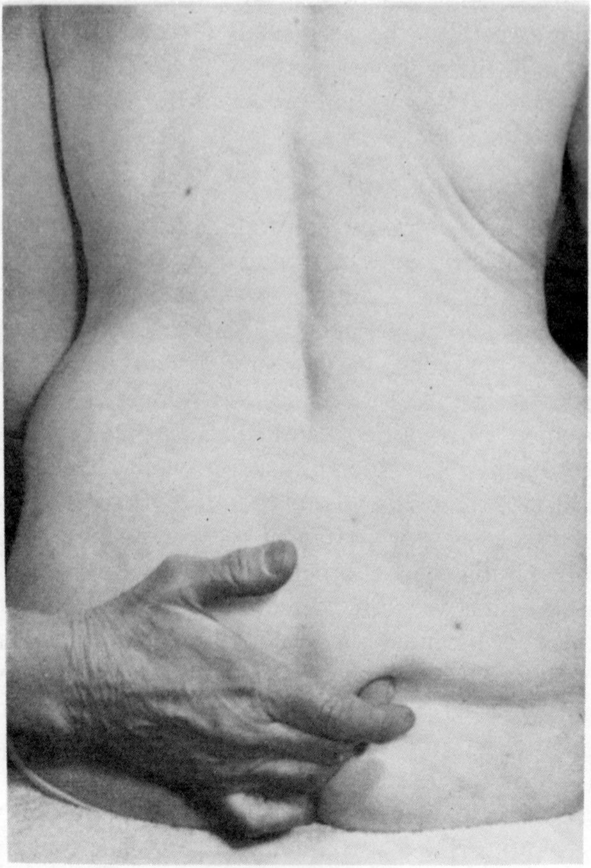

FIG. 13
Stroking technique.
Position of hand and fingers applying tension.

the whole body surface. This is very important in the treatment of all types of headache. During a discussion with the patient existing " silent " zones such as a liver zone may disclose the original cause of the headaches. Normalization of the liver zone will therefore improve the symptomatic condition of headache. Concentration on headache zones alone would not produce a satisfactory result.

Manual Technique of Massage

The effective stimulus to produce results with C.T.M. is probably a specific movement carried out by the fingers of the operator's hand, resulting in alteration of the tension of cutaneous and subcutaneous tissue. Some American authors (Behrend 1954) describe it as subdermal traction. This is a very good description of the effect which must be produced by the movement of the fingers and will avoid faulty manipulations. The beginner is inclined to use too much pressure which nails the surface tissues down and therefore prevents movement between tissue layers or movement between surface tissues and subcutaneous tissues. Another fault which sometimes occurs is movement between the fingers of the operator and the skin of the patient producing a frictional movement which results in a haematoma. Haematoma is produced by injury to small capillary vessels resulting in blood-release into the neighbouring tissue. This must be absorbed speedily or it will lead to formation of scar tissue. The tensile stimulus is most frequently carried out by using the middle finger supported by the ring finger producing a stroking movement. The operator touches the patient's skin to obtain adherence either with the radial side of the palmar surface of the terminal phalanx of the middle finger or the surface area of the finger tip. (Short nails.) The choice will be influenced by the treated area. (Fig. 13)

The increase in tension is produced by movement of the superficial on the deeper tissues, *i.e.*, the cutaneous on the subcutaneous tissue or on the fascial layer. Tension may also be increased in interstitial tissue by applying the strokes along intermuscular septa or along the borders of aponeurosis. This tensile stimulus is produced by obtaining a certain adherence of the finger tip on the skin. Lubricants must therefore never be used on the operator's hands or the patient's skin. The next step is to take up the slack of the superficial tissue, and thirdly to continue in the direction of the movement. For the beginner it is helpful to concentrate on the following movement sequence. Touch firmly, take up the slack, pull. Pressure which exceeds the necessary amount for adherence is detrimental to the effectiveness of the massage. It diminishes the possibilities of increased tissue tension. Healthy tissue passes as a fluent fold in front of the moving finger. A real resistance may be encountered by the moving finger due to the adherence of superficial on deep tissue. The finger must never be forced through the tissue. If great resistance is encountered, it is advisable to use a shorter, lifting stroke. The tissues become gradually more mobile. The fingers touch the skin at an angle of approximately 45°. This angle may be altered to make the massage more or less deep. Decrease of the angle will decrease the depth; increase of the angle will increase the depth. The amount of sensation can be adjusted by modifying the speed of the stroke. The slower movement will decrease the sensation. Adherence of the finger-tip can be obtained by touching the skin with either the radial side or the middle of the palmar surface of the finger-tip, depending on the area under treatment. The radial side of the wrist joint or its anterior aspect must lead the movement. The latter is particularly important in the application of short lifting strokes. This also permits use of the elbow flexors and so avoids harmful strain on the interphalangeal joints, especially the terminal joint and the intrinsic muscles of the hand.

At the impact of the finger-tips on the skin, the patient must have no other sensation than that of touch. Should a scratching or cutting sensation already be felt at that moment, the technique should be revised. It is possible to exert too much initial pull or touch the patient's skin with the finger-nails which must always be kept very short.

Direction of stroke

In the paravertebral areas the stroke follows on the whole the direction of the dermatomes. In the periphery it follows the direction of muscle fibres (*e.g.*, deltoid), muscle fascia (*e.g.*, bicipital fascia, ilio-tibial tract), tendons (*e.g.*, tendo achillis) or it passes at right angles to intermuscular septa (*e.g.*, the septum dividing the anterior from the lateral compartment in the calf), or at right angles to fascial borders (*e.g.*, along the border of latissimus dorsi).

The following diagrams show the important fascial structures, muscle borders and tendons.

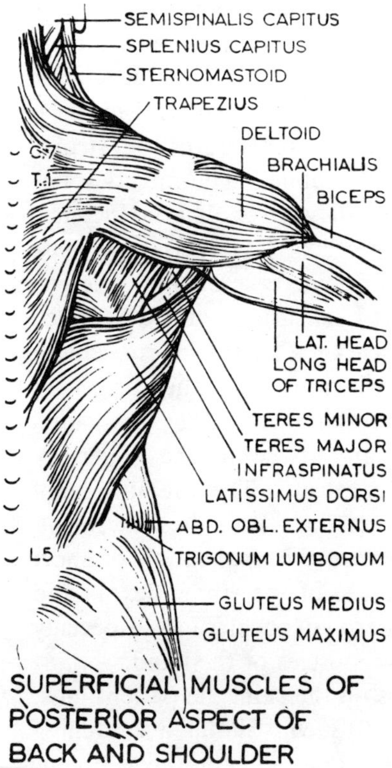

SUPERFICIAL MUSCLES OF POSTERIOR ASPECT OF BACK AND SHOULDER

FIG. 14

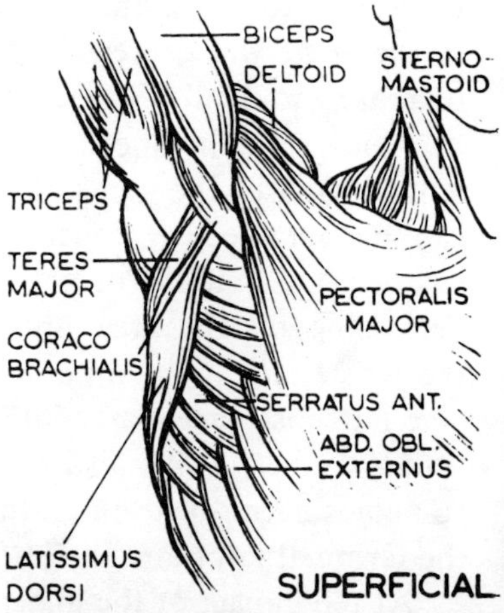

SUPERFICIAL MUSCLES OF AXILLA, CHEST, NECK AND ARM.

FIG. 15

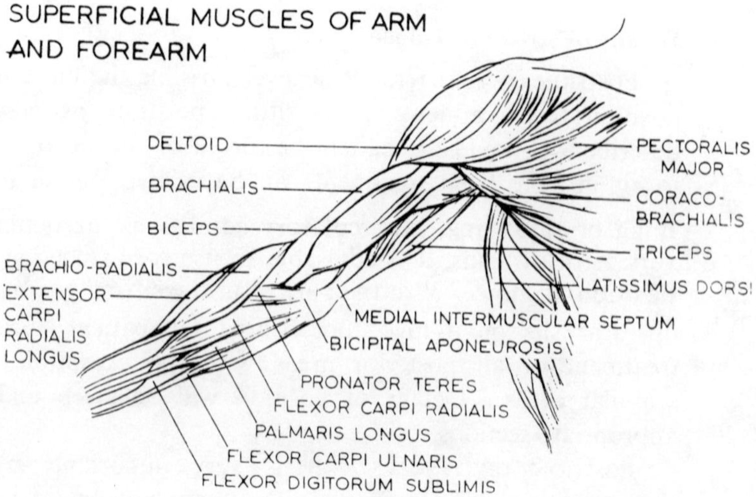

FIG. 16

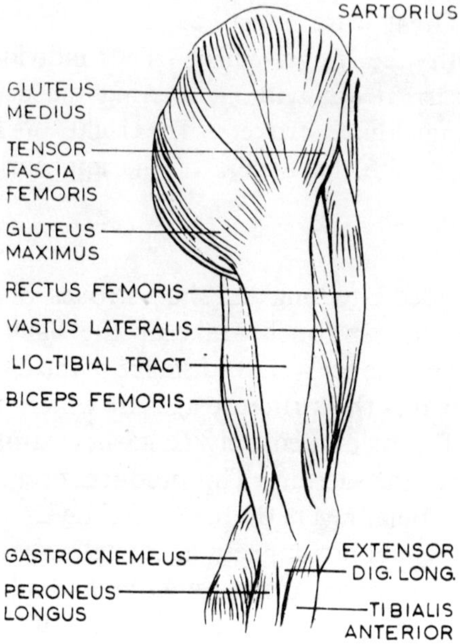

SUPERFICIAL MUSCLES OF THE LATERAL ASPECT OF THE THIGH

FIG. 17

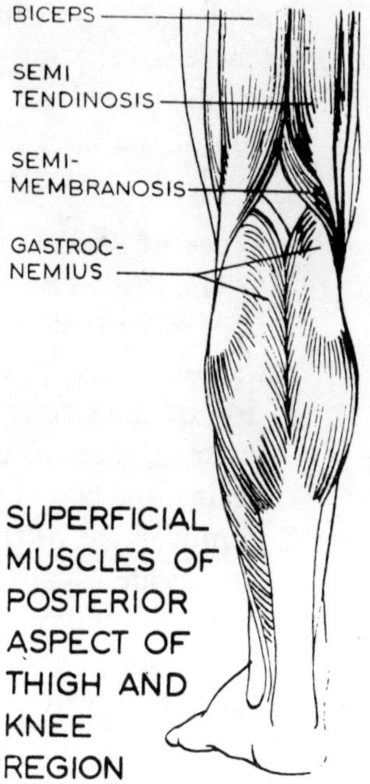

FIG. 18

Details of stroke technique

POSITION OF PATIENT. Whenever possible the most suitable position for treatment is the sitting position, as previously described. Should the patient be too ill or too uncomfortable to sit up, the back treatment can be carried out in forward lying or side lying. In circulatory conditions, particularly in varicosity of veins, it is advisable to use forward lying as the position of choice. With the patient in the sitting position, the operator sits on a low stool behind the patient during the treatment of all posterior areas with the exception of the scapular areas. Details of position will be given under the appropriate sections.

POSITION OF FINGERS. It is very important to touch the patient's skin very firmly without applying more pressure than is necessary to create a condition of adherence between finger-tips and skin. Great care must be taken not to apply any pressure with the finger-nails. The individual tensile stroke must be carried out without altering the depth or the speed of the individual stroke. The right or left side of the back is treated with the fingers of the appropriate hand.

Types of stroke

The strokes may be divided into long and short strokes. Short strokes consist of three phases: Touch—take up the slack of the superficial tissues—continue for a short distance in the direction of the stroke until it hits the structure against which it is directed, then lift up the fingers immediately. (E.g. short strokes against the lateral border of the sacrum.) This produces primarily movement of the superficial layers on the fascial layer. The strokes are usually directed at approximately right angles against bone, muscular or fascial borders or indurated areas such as scar tissue. They are more localised in their effect and are less likely to cause unexpected widespread reaction.

Long strokes are identical in the first two phases with the short strokes but then continue with the working fingers at the achieved depth, letting a small fold of skin run along of them with the aim of producing free movement between the superficial and deeper layers. Long strokes very often follow the original cleavage lines (*e.g.* costal strokes, Fig. 40) or pass along fascial borders (*e.g.* along ilio-tibial tract, Fig. 34).

On no account must the fingers be forced through the tissues. Adherent areas must be freed by short lifting strokes.

TREATMENT AREAS. The back is divided for treatment purposes into sections. The details of the stroke technique will be described under the headings of Basic Section, Thoracic Section and Cervical Section. The headings of all other treatment sections are self-explanatory.

Basic section

This includes the sacral and lumbar areas including T.12 and the subcostal stroke.

The treatment usually begins with short strokes, approximately 1 to 1½ inches long (Fig. 19) which are carried at right angles to the lateral border of the sacrum and towards the line of the sacro-iliac joint. The flexor surface or the radial side of the finger-tip is usually in contact with the patient's skin. Short lifting strokes are carried out. Should the tension between subcutaneous tissue and fascia be very great, it may be advisable to use the palmar surface of the finger-tip to decrease the cutting sensation. Once free movement of the superficial on the deeper tissues is obtained, a long stroke is carried from the widest part of the sacrum towards the anal cleft.

Short lifting strokes are carried out next at right angles towards the iliac crest, using the radial or palmar part of the finger-tips depending on the existing basic tension.

Short tensile strokes are next carried into the angle between the posterior superior iliac spine and the transverse process of L.5. The first stroke runs almost parallel to the iliac crest, passing from lateral to medial. The following two or three strokes pass slightly steeper into the sacro-lumbar angle until the last stroke passes almost vertically down into the angle space. Strokes are repeated approx. 3-10 times.

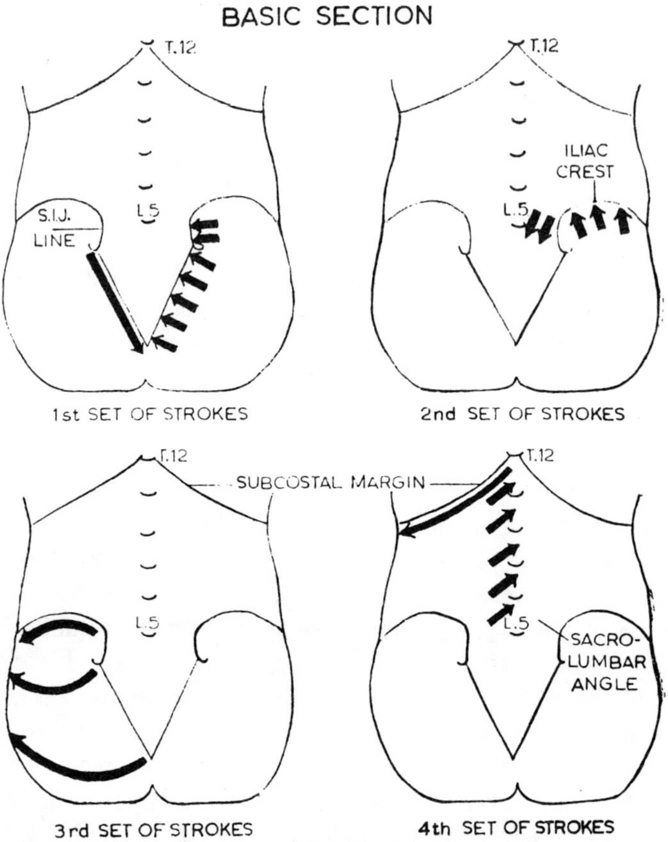

FIG. 19

Once the tension in the sacral and pelvic area has improved three long strokes are carried over the ilium. The first stroke passes close to the iliac crest, starting at the transverse process of L.5 towards the anterior superior iliac spine, where it is terminated with a short lifting movement round the spine, carrying the stroke a short distance backwards above the iliac crest.

The second stroke starts at the widest part of the sacrum, passes laterally and forward, aiming for the anterior superior iliac spine and terminating in the same manner as the first stroke.

The third stroke starts at the anal cleft and passes forward above the great trochanter to terminate in the same way as the previously described strokes.

The sacral region contains tension areas in most people but particularly in patients who are obliged to stand for long periods. It is therefore very important to pay particular attention to exact technique. Skin friction or deep pressure may produce faulty reactions such as sudden headaches, irritating skin sensation over the homolateral thigh, sometimes even as high up as the axilla, or over the contralateral thigh. It is very important to deal with these reactions at once. Very often application of correct tensile strokes over the sacrum and particularly the iliac crest area will quickly relieve the faulty reactions. Should this be unsuccessful it will be necessary to treat at once the great trochanter area of the femur on its posterior side, followed by strokes along the iliac crest.

The basic section is completed with approximately five short strokes which are carried from lateral to medial over the erector spinae area following the space between the transverse processes of the lumbar vertebrae. These strokes are so short that it is difficult to get phase 3 in without touching the spinous processes of the lumbar vertebrae. It has therefore proved practical to get the final tension by slightly turning the fingers cranialwards in a lifting movement. The final stroke of this section is carried from medial to lateral following the lower border of the thoracic cage. In carrying out this stroke, as well as the pelvic strokes, it is very important to hold the hand in such a position that the radial part of the wrist is leading. This will result in the correct tensile stimulus on the tissues.

Flat-handed release strokes over the anterior aspect of the trunk are usually appreciated by the patient before terminating a basic section treatment. These are carried out with both hands flat, starting over the anterior midline of the trunk, and simultaneously being carried backwards and laterally to terminate approximately in the mid-axillary line. The hands should be well moulded over the body surface.

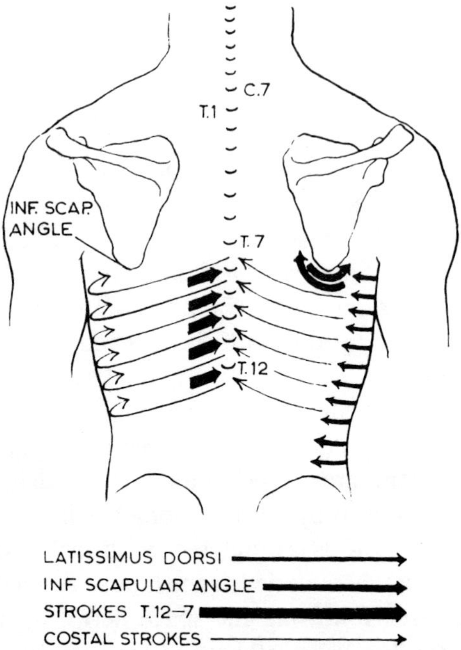

THORACIC SECTION 1.

FIG. 20

Thoracic section

This includes the areas from T.12 to T.1 and the costal areas as far as the inferior angle of the scapula. It also includes the treatment of the lateral border of latissimus dorsi as far as the axilla. The latissimus dorsi may have to be treated before the erector spinae areas close to the thoracic vertebral spines, especially if the patient shows visceral reactions such as dyspnoea, or palpitations. The whole of the thoracic area involves stimulation of preganglionic fibres. It is therefore advisable to intersperse the treatment of this section with anterior release strokes. Adverse visceral reactions can be relieved by returning to the pelvic section and if necessary treating the great trochanter area. The treatment of this section demands particular care. Should it be difficult to obtain the scratching or cutting reaction, it is advisable

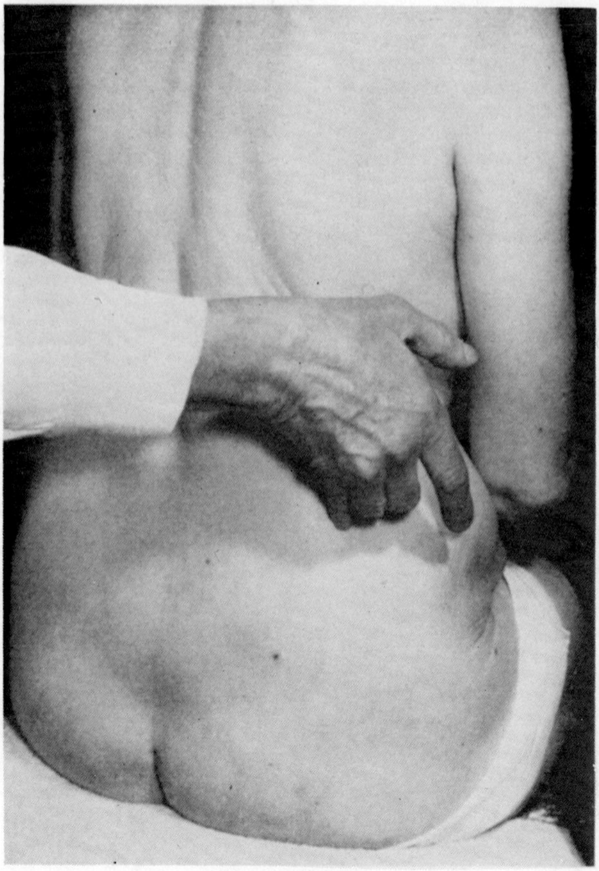

FIG. 21

Stroking technique.

Position of hand at the beginning of iliac crest stroke.

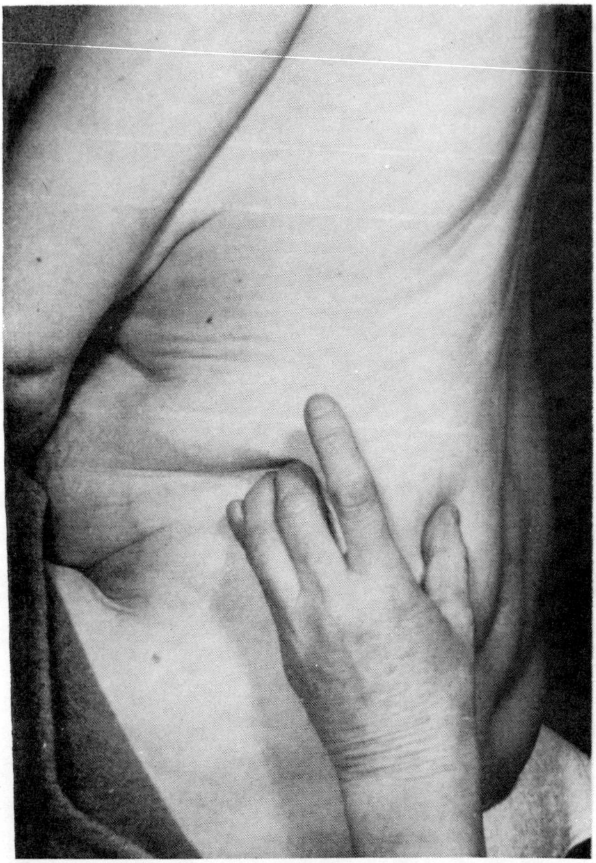

FIG. 22

Stroking technique.

Position of hand at the end of iliac crest stroke.

to treat the latissimus dorsi borders. Should it be difficult to obtain a satisfactory reaction from this area, it is essential to return to the basic section. The stimulation of the paravertebral areas from T.7 to T.1 should not be attempted before tension areas over the scapulae have started to clear up and a clear cutting sensation is obtained in these areas.

Latissimus dorsi

It is essential to obtain a clear picture of the lateral border of latissimus dorsi by asking the patient to carry out a resisted adduction movement, starting from the shoulder level position of the upper arm.

The palmar surface of the finger-tips of the homolateral hand are placed at the border of latissimus dorsi and a short tensile stroke is carried from lateral to medial, almost placing the finger-tips under the lateral border of the muscle. A sharp cutting reaction is usually obtained easily with correct technique. The strokes start at the iliac crest and are carried in short intervals to the axillary border of the muscle. At the level of T.7 the inferior angle of the scapulae should be included in the stimulation. The finger-tips are placed just below the inferior scapular angle, slightly to the lateral side of the angle with sufficient pressure to make them adherent to the skin. The latter usually shows great mobility in that area. The whole tissue is then carried by the finger-tips from the lateral border of the angle round the apex up the medial border of the angle. This easily produces the tensile stimulus. Should it be difficult to obtain the cutting reaction over the latissimus dorsi border, this manipulation will help to obtain the correct reaction (Fig. 20).

T.12 to T.7

Short lifting strokes are carried over the erector spinae area from lateral to medial, following the space between the transverse processes of the lower thoracic vertebrae, and ending with the same lifting action as previously described.

Costal strokes

These follow the direction of the previously described subcostal stroke along the intercostal spaces. At first the stroke starts in the mid-axillary line and is carefully carried backwards towards the vertebral column. These strokes are usually very cutting and the fingers should therefore be placed at a fairly acute angle. At subsequent treatment sessions when the sensation becomes less acute, it is possible to carry the stroke in both directions, starting at the vertebral end of the intercostal space in the same manner as the iliac crest stroke, passing forward to approximately the lateral vertical plane, turning carefully round and passing backwards to the starting point (Fig. 20).

Scapular region

For the treatment as described in the following paragraph the operator stands at right angles to the patient's thorax on the side of the scapula to be treated. The treatment is carried out with the contralateral hand, *e.g.*, the right scapula with the left hand. The first set of strokes consists of short lifting strokes, passing from the inferior angle of the scapula along its vertebral border to its superior angle. This is followed by a long stroke along the whole of the medial border. The next stroke passes from the inferior angle of the scapula along the lateral border towards the axilla. It will be found that it is advisable to hold the fingers at a very acute angle for this stroke as tension is often very great. The infraspinous and supraspinous fossae are treated with short lifting strokes passing at right angles towards the scapular spine. This set of strokes is completed by passing a long stroke along the superior border of the scapular spine, starting from the root of the spine and stroking towards the acromion process, letting the angle of the stroking finger get more acute as it nears the tip of the shoulder. A set of strokes is then carried out passing from medial to lateral, converging to the axilla and gradually filling the whole of the infraspinous fossa, so that the last stroke passes along the inferior border of the scapular spine. In cases of high tissue tension (*e.g.*, periarthritis of the shoulder joint) it may not be possible to treat the infraspinous fossa until the paravertebral areas from T.6 to the occiput have been normalized in tension. This particularly applies if trigger points (Travell, 1951) exist in the infraspinous fossa. In these cases it may prove beneficial to apply short lifting strokes in the infraspinous fossa, along the medial scapular border starting from lateral to medial. These strokes are carried out by the homolateral hand, with the operator standing behind the patient.

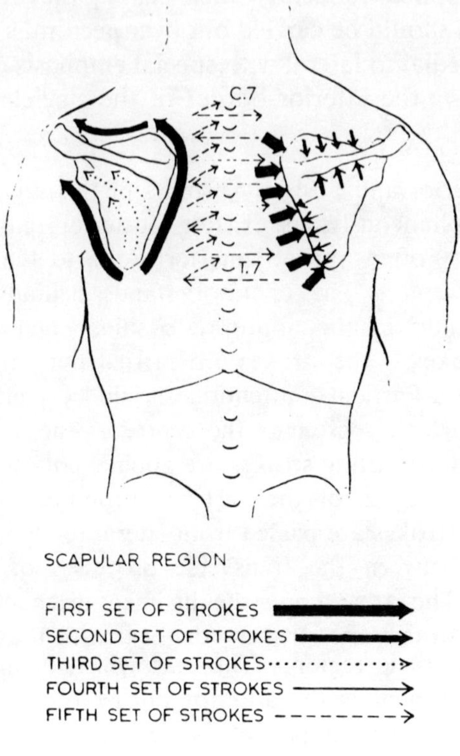

THORACIC SECTION 2.

FIG. 23

Thoracic spine T.6 to T.1

Short lifting strokes are passed from lateral to medial, following the spaces between the transverse processes of the upper thoracic vertebrae. In all cases of increased tissue tension in this area (*e.g.*, headaches of various origin) it proves advisable to treat this area intensively with transverse strokes which are carried out with alternate hands, passing across the region between the scapulae, carefully stroking through the intervals below the thoracic spinous processes. A change to the border of the tip of the treating finger proves useful. Anterior release strokes should be applied frequently when treating the thoracic region. The strokes should be carried out over pectoralis major, passing from medial to lateral with special emphasis on the stroke passing along the inferior border of the clavicle (Fig. 23).

Cervical region

The anterior and posterior aspects of this region should be treated simultaneously, as existing posterior tension areas, if relieved, very often appear anteriorly due to the structure of the fascial septa. The operator stands behind the patient, moving slightly to the appropriate side, when carrying out anterior strokes. The strokes are carried out with the homolateral hand. Particular attention should be paid to the area round C.7 which represents the centre of the aponeurosis of trapezius. Short lifting strokes are applied converging towards the spinous process of the vertebra prominens. Thereafter, short lifting strokes are passed from lateral to medial, following the spaces between the transverse processes of the cervical vertebrae. The area along the ligamentum nuchae is again treated with transverse strokes, identical with those applied to the upper thoracic region. The part which in many patients demands treatment is the anterior border of trapezius. This particularly applies to patients suffering from headaches or circulatory disturbances of the upper limb. The anterior border of the upper section of trapezius is treated in a manner similar to the lateral border of latissimus dorsi. Short lifting strokes are applied at right angles along the border, right up to the attachment on the curved line of the occiput. This is followed by a long stroke, passing along the border of the muscle, applying traction with a slight steadying action of the contralateral hand on the head.

Anteriorly the floor of the posterior triangle of the neck is covered with short strokes, passing from the clavicular base of the triangle cranialward tos its apex. The posterior border of the sternomastoid is followed to its attachment on the mastoid process. These strokes are interspersed with strokes following the superior and inferior borders of the clavicle.

Should it be difficult to obtain satisfactory reaction to any of the above described strokes, it usually proves helpful to pay particular attention to the tissues in the triangle enclosed by the acromion process and the posterior border of the clavicle. A short sharp tensile stroke is applied, directed towards the apex of this triangular area (Figs. 24, 25).

Shoulder and upper arm region

With the exception of severe circulatory disturbances such as occur in A.P.M. and angiospastic disturbances, *e.g.*, Raynaud's disease, it is very rarely necessary to progress beyond the treatment as described in this section. In all conditions affecting the shoulder joint or the periarticular structures involving the function of the joint, it is essential to have treated the back at least to the level of T.12, the latissimus dorsi, and the scapular and cervical regions. In most cases the treatment of these areas will already have given great symptomatic relief of paraesthetic or neuralgic complaints. For a final clearing up of all symptoms including restriction of movements (unless this is due to severe articular destruction) it is advisable to include the treatment of the areas described below. The treatment strokes for latissimus dorsi and trapezius have already been described. Before encroaching on the line of the shoulder joint itself, it is advisable to treat the pectoral and deltoid regions.

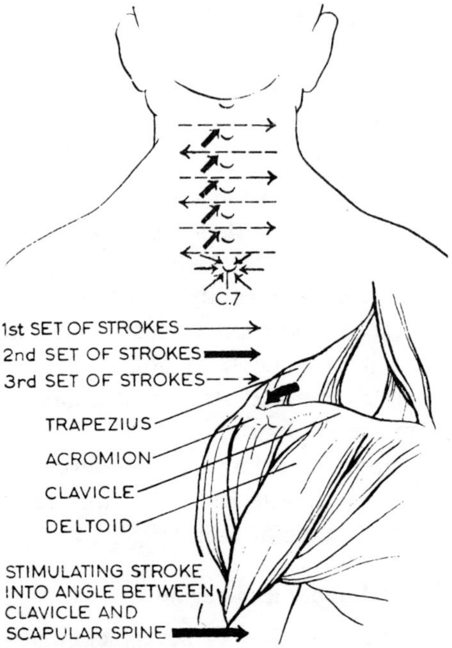

FIG. 24
Cervical region.
Posterior aspect.

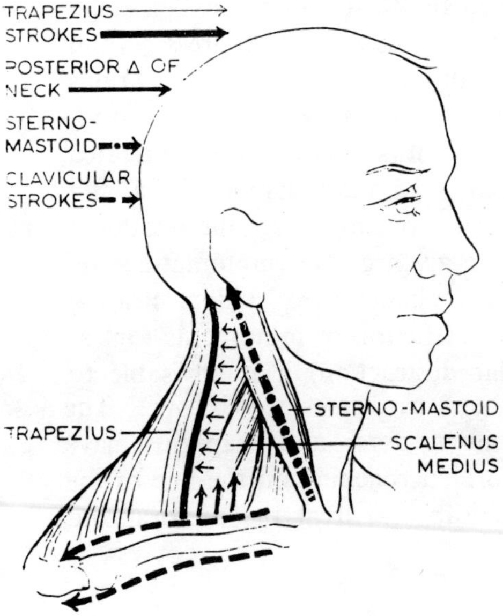

FIG. 25
Cervical region.
Lateral aspect.

Pectoral region

This has been previously approached when giving release strokes in a flat-handed manner during the treatment of the back regions. It can now be included with deeper subcutaneous strokes, passing from the lateral border of the sternum converging towards the axillary space. The strokes along the superior and inferior border of the clavicle are also included in the treatment of this section.

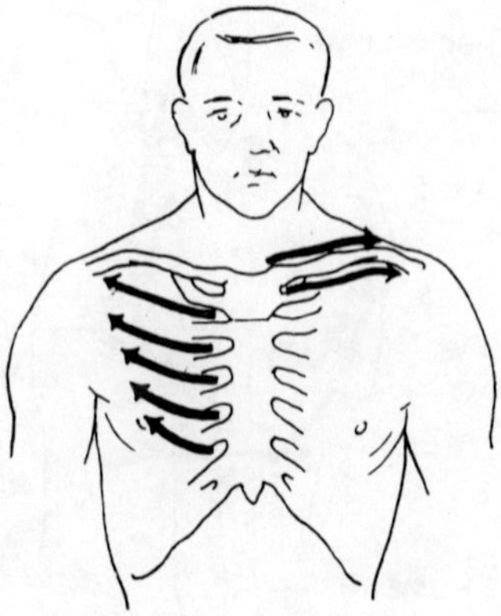

PECTORAL REGION

FIG. 26

Deltoid region

The physiotherapist stands at right angles to the patient on the homolateral side. The arm to be treated should be supported in slight abduction in order to allow movement of the superficial on the deeper tissues.

The posterior margin of the right deltoid is treated with the left hand, while the right hand supports the arm. In order to treat the anterior margin of deltoid the hands change places. Short lifting strokes are applied at right angles to the anterior and posterior margins of the muscle, starting from the scapular and the clavicular attachment of the muscle respectively and progressing towards the humeral insertion. In all cases of periarthritis of the shoulder it is advisable to add strokes along the intermuscular septa of the deltoid origin from the acromion process. It is very important to pay particular attention to the scratching or cutting reaction which indicates a satisfactory circulatory reaction. Should the patient report only a pressure sensation, it is essential to return to the treatment of the scapula. *i.e.*, stimulation of the angle between scapular spine and clavicle as previously described. A short stimulating stroke, carried out in the subclavian triangle towards the clavicle often helps to obtain a satisfactory reaction as it probably causes a direct

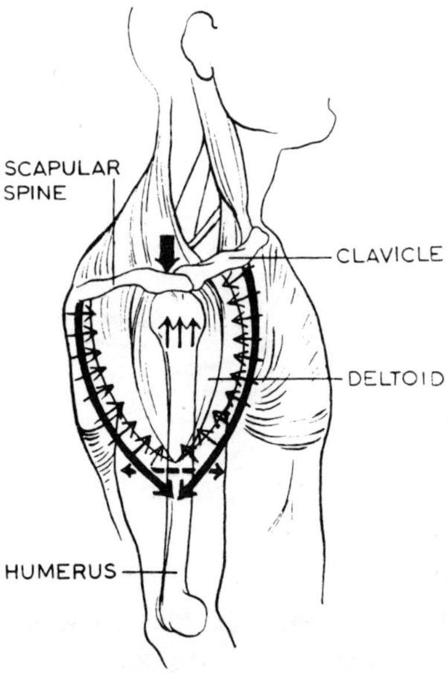

DELTOID REGION Lateral view.

FIG. 27

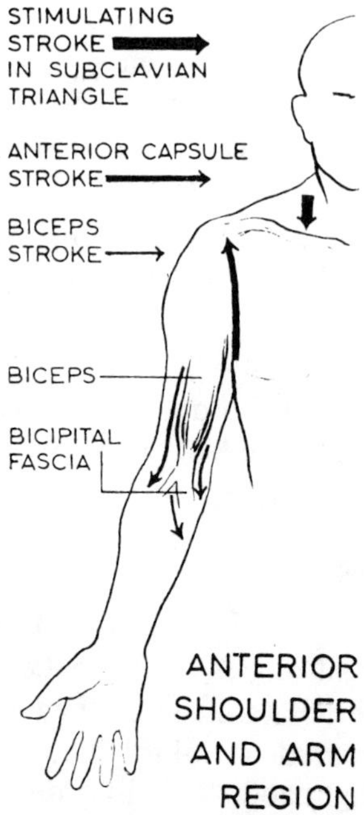

FIG. 28

stimulation of the subclavian vessels. The deltoid area is completed by stroking along the contour of the muscle anteriorly and posteriorly from origin to insertion, finishing with small transverse strokes across the insertion.

The next strokes cover the attachments of the capsule of the shoulder joint, starting at the axilla and leading anteriorly and posteriorly upwards towards the superior extremity of the joint.

The biceps is treated in particular in its distal part. Long strokes are carried along the medial and lateral borders of the biceps tendon into the lateral compartment of the antecubital fossa. The final biceps stroke is taken medially along the border of the bicipital fascia. This stroke is usually very sharp and must therefore be made carefully. It is one of the most important strokes in this area. Paraesthesia in the hands is often relieved by this stroke.

Forearm and hand

In many cases it will not be necessary to treat these areas because pain and circulatory symptoms will have disappeared while treating the back and cervical regions. In the presence of trophic disturbances (*e.g.*, A.P.M.) and peripheral circulatory diseases (intermittent claudication) it may occasionally be necessary to treat the peripheral parts. In most patients peripheral symptoms will have disappeared by improving the more proximally situated part of the circulation.

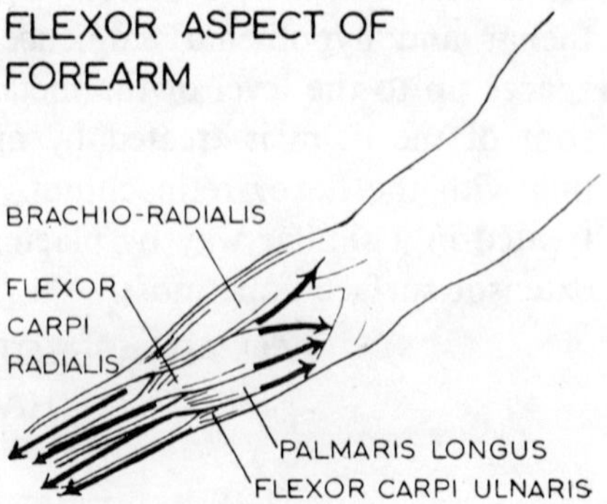

FIG. 29

FOREARM. As the major vessels lie anteriorly, only the anterior part of the forearm is treated. Four strokes are applied from distal to proximal, *i.e.*, towards the antecubital fossa: laterally along the border of brachioradialis and flexor carpi radialis, medially along the borders of the palmaris longus (if present), and along flexor carpi ulnaris. The more distally situated part of these regions is treated by starting the stroke in the middle of the forearm and completing it in the direction of the wrist joint. Should it be necessary to treat the posterior aspect of the forearm, the strokes are applied to the borders of extensor digitorum communis. For all these strokes the elbow is held in the semi-flexed position.

WRIST. Short strokes are applied from proximal to distal along the palmar tendons. The same type of strokes are applied on the dorsal aspect of the wrist region along the extensor tendons.

The hand is held in the neutral position for the application of these strokes. Should it be difficult to obtain the cutting sensation it may prove helpful to place the fingers firmly along the tendon border, take up the slack of the superficial tissue until the fingers become arrested, and then move the patient's hand quickly into extension when applying palmar strokes and into flexion when applying strokes on the extensor surface.

HAND. The palm of the hand is treated by placing it flat on a soft but firm surface. Strokes are applied along the thenar and hypothenar eminence and along the interosseous spaces up to the level of the metacarpophalangeal joints. The root of the palm is treated by applying transverse strokes in line with the flexor retinaculum. The dorsum of the hand is treated in a similar way by placing the patient's hand with the extensor surface uppermost.

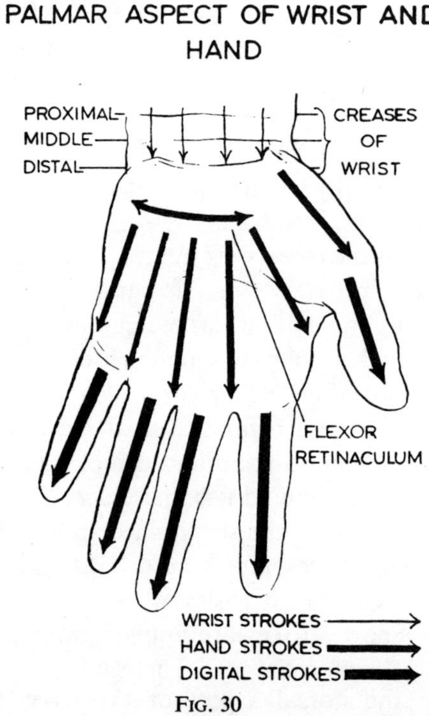

FIG. 30

FINGERS. Only the palmar surface of the fingers is treated. The patient places the hand, palm downwards, on the hand of the operator who strokes from the base of the fingers towards the finger-tip. If these strokes prove difficult, stroking along the lateral border of the finger may help. (*E.g.* scleroderma.)

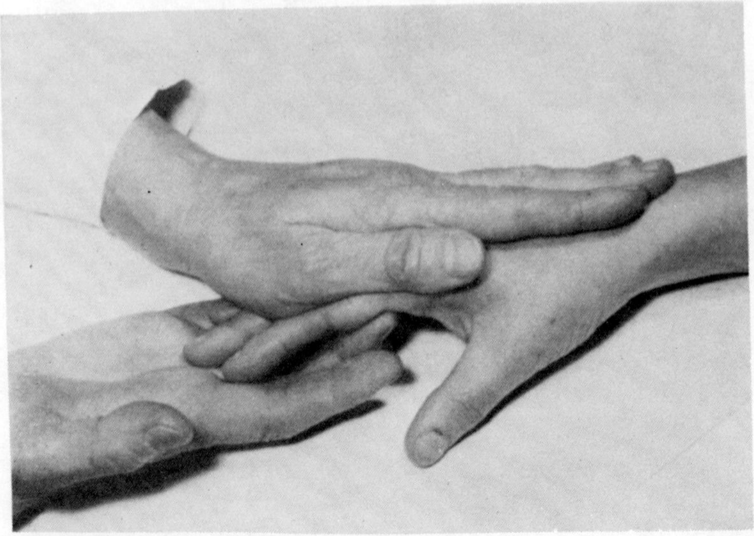

FIG. 31

Stroking technique.

Position of hands during digital strokes.

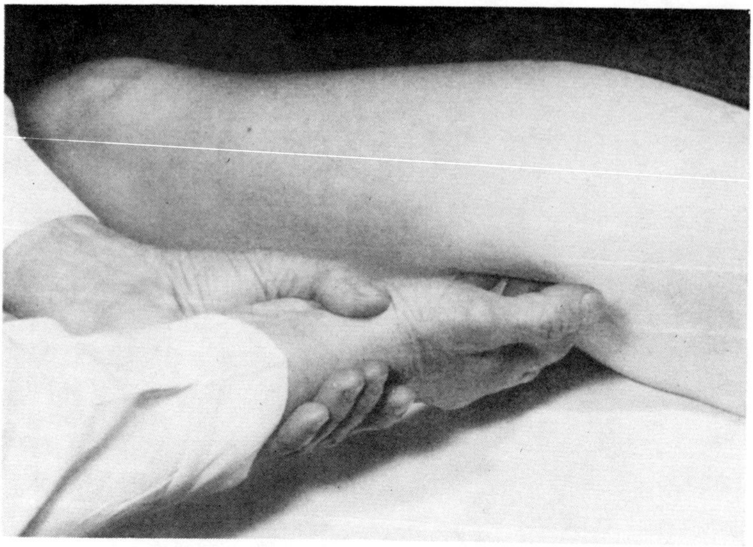

Fig. 32

Stroking technique.

Wrist support for the working hand during iliotibial tract strokes.

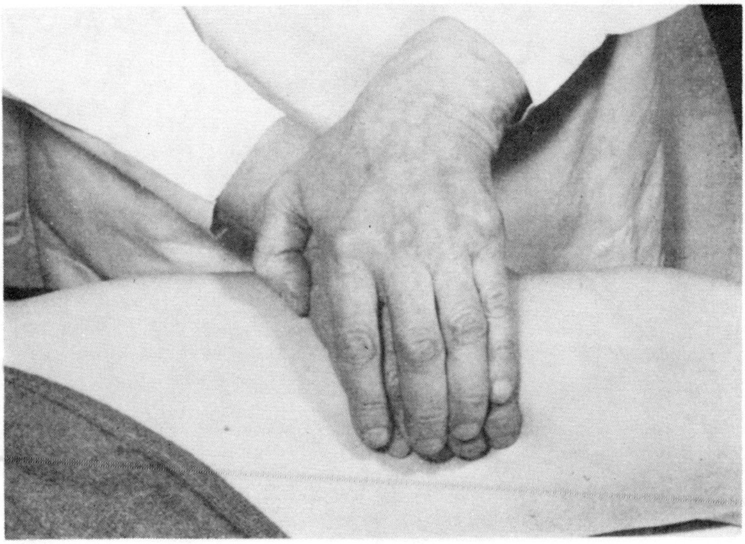

Fig. 33

Stimulation of adductor hiatus trigger point.

Femoral region

This is one of the most important regions for treatment, as muscular and fascial structures are to a great extent continuous with those of the pelvic region. In man the circulation in the lower limb is particularly vulnerable, especially those in occupations which involve long periods of standing. In standing the muscular pump is to a great extent out of action and as a result of this the fascial structures become thickened and tend to shorten. This applies particularly to the iliotibial tract which receives the whole of the insertion of tensor fascia femoris and part of the insertion of gluteus maximus. These two muscles are held contracted during standing, and tend to shorten the iliotibial tract. A stagnant peripheral circulation must invariably influence the more proximal part of the circulation. This explains why it is often necessary to treat the upper femoral region before it is possible to obtain satisfactory results over the pelvic region. The femoral vessels become twice superficial in the femoral region (femoral triangle, adductor hiatus) and it is therefore comparatively easy to stimulate the circulation. All treatments of this region should be carried out with the patient in the lying position. Should this prove impossible the side lying position may prove acceptable to the patient. In this case the knee of the lower leg should be comfortably bent, and a pillow placed between the two legs to allow steady positioning of the upper leg. The treatment of the iliotibial tract often proves very fatiguing for the hand of the operator. Under such conditions it proves helpful to support the wrist of the working hand with other hand.

UPPER FEMORAL REGION. The most important part of this region is the iliotibial tract and the great trochanter area. Short lifting strokes are applied at right angles to the posterior margin of the tract, beginning approximately in the middle of the thigh and working upwards in short intervals towards the great trochanter. These strokes may be experienced by the

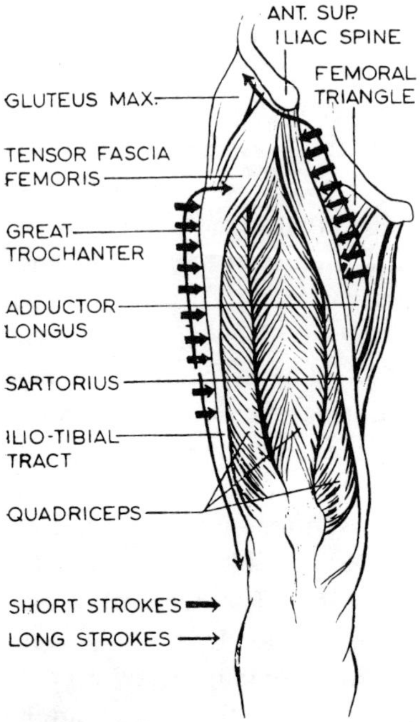

ANTERIOR
THIGH REGION

Fig. 34

patient as very sharp and the amount of tensile stimulation must therefore be varied carefully. It is essential to obtain a correct sensory reaction from the patient as otherwise skin irritations may appear over the whole of the limb. Should the patient report these faulty reactions, it is wise to pay particular attention to the correct application of technique. Should the second attempt still produce a faulty reaction, the circulation may be stimulated from a *trigger point* over the *adductor hiatus*. To apply this stimulating stroke, the operator stands on the homolateral side and places the fingers over the adductor hiatus, resting the hand over the anterior aspect of the thigh with the dorsum of the hand uppermost. In order to make the fingers more adaptable it sometimes proves useful to steady the hand by resting the other hand on top. The patient should be warned beforehand of the extremely sharp, almost electrical shock sensation resulting from this very short stimulating stroke (Fig. 33). After the short strokes applied along the upper portion of the iliotibial tract, a long stroke is passed along the tract passing from distal to proximal and ending round the great trochanter.

The sartorius region is treated in its upper part in a similar way to the upper part of the iliotibial tract. The operator stands on the homolateral side and applies short strokes at right angles along the medial border of the muscle which forms the lateral boundary of the femoral triangle. These short strokes are followed by a long stroke from the middle of the thigh towards the anterior superior iliac spine where the stroke is terminated round the spine for a short distance, following the iliac crest. The lower regions of the thigh are stimulated by stroking laterally along the distal part of the iliotibial tract, starting in the middle of the thigh and terminating at the level of the knee joint. A similar stroke is applied along the border of biceps. Medially a stroke is applied between semimembranosus and semitendinosus, both strokes terminating at the level of the knee joint.

Posterior Aspect of the Thigh

In a number of conditions of circulatory disturbance in the lower limb, it will prove necessary to stimulate the vessels derived from deep branches of the femoral artery affecting the hamstring area. In these cases the patient is placed into the forward lying position with a pillow under the abdomen, supporting the lumbar spine. It is usually possible to use long strokes, starting in the middle of the thigh and carrying approximately 3-4 strokes upwards towards the gluteus maximus area covering the upper hamstring area. The lower hamstring area is covered following the lower parts of biceps fem., semi-tendinosis and semi-membranosis.

Knee and leg region

In most patients the circulatory and paraesthetic symptoms will have cleared up during the treatment of the previously described regions. It might, however, be necessary to treat the whole of the lower leg for conditions as mentioned under hand region. In some cases of trauma in the region of the knee joint, the treatment of the knee region proves useful in order to improve the movement range if it should be difficult to obtain maximum possible joint movement by exercise therapy alone. This applies particularly to conditions where scar tissue or adhesions are present.

KNEE REGION. Short lifting strokes are applied, converging on the patella. The stroke parallel with the joint line often proves painful and should therefore be omitted. Special attention should be paid to the medial and lateral vastus retinaculae on either side of the ligamentum patellae. It may not be possible to obtain a satisfactory reaction to the strokes along the superior and inferior margins of the patella, and these are better omitted under such conditions (Fig. 35).

Posteriorly two strokes are applied, starting at the meeting point of the two heads of gastrocnemius, passing towards the popliteal space, and diverging towards the medial and lateral femoral condyles. Laterally a series of short strokes may be applied if symptoms are concentrated over the peroneal and lateral malleolar areas. The patient's leg is held in semi-flexion with the foot resting on the plinth. The operator sits on the homolateral side facing the patient. The operator's hand is applied to the patient's calf in the same way as a hand would hold the neck of a violin, so that the fingers come to rest easily in the groove between the lateral head of gastrocnemius and peroneus longus. Short tensile strokes are carried out over an area of two to three inches starting at the fibular end of the groove and applying the tensile stimulation in the direction from the anterior to the posterior margins of the lateral aspect of the leg (Fig. 36).

Should it be difficult to obtain a satisfactory reaction, it will prove helpful to give one or two short stimulating strokes at the meeting point of the two heads of gastrocnemius with soleus. The hand lies with the palm applied to the calf, the fingers pointing upwards. The stroke is carried in the direction towards the heel but is very short. The patient should again be warned before this trigger area is stimulated. The reaction may be very sharp (Fig. 37).

A stroke on either side of the tendo achillis is applied bimanually, starting at the level of the beginning of the tendon and stroking from proximal to distal.

In order to synchronize all the stimuli given over small regions in the lower extremity, it will be advisable to terminate

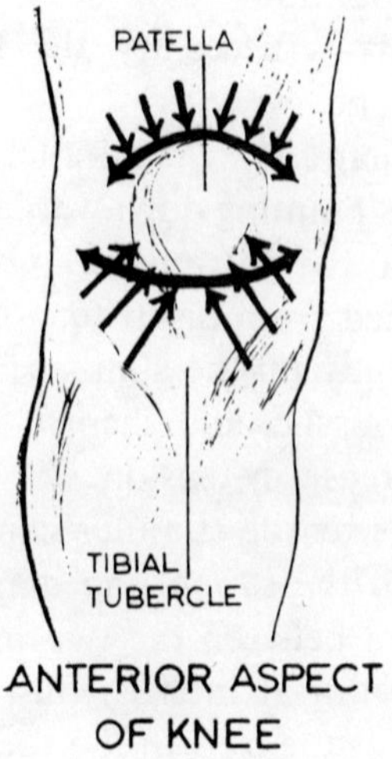

FIG. 35

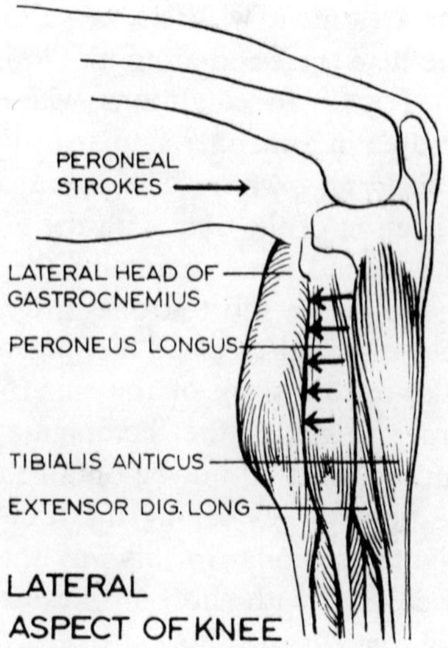

FIG. 36

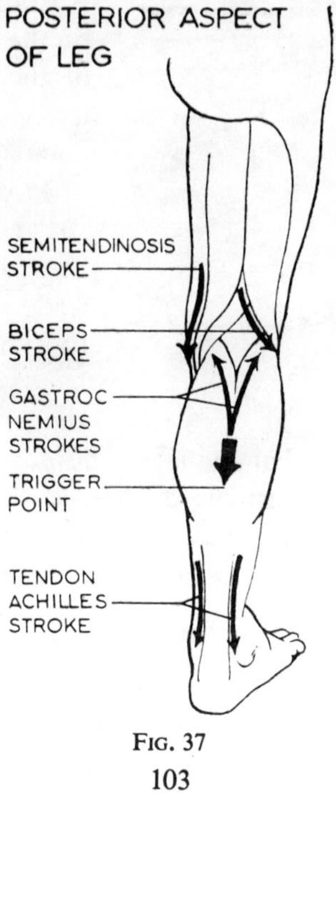

FIG. 37

the treatment with strokes along the iliotibial tract and over the iliac crest and along the long saphenous vein.

FOOT. In conditions where this is necessary the foot is treated in a manner similar to the hand.

Dorsal aspect. The operator's hand is held parallel to the direction of the tibia with the fingers pointing downwards, while the second hand maintains the foot at right angles. Over the ankle region short strokes are applied from distal to proximal. It is essential to place the fingers firmly on the skin surface, to take up the slack of the superficial tissue, and then to pull in order to obtain the therapeutic increase in tension. Should a cutting reaction not be obtained, the tensile stimulus can again be obtained by taking the foot with the supporting hand into plantar flexion. In this way the area between the two malleoli is covered with short strokes. The dorsal interosseous spaces are treated with short strokes as far as the cleft of the toes.

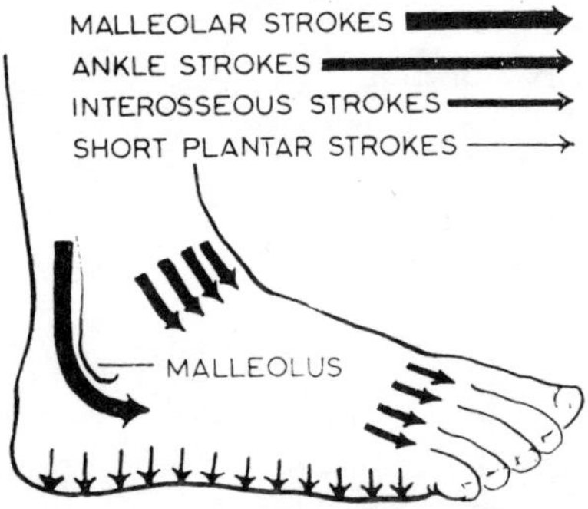

FIG. 38
Dorsal aspect of foot.

Medial and lateral aspects. A stroke is placed, starting on the medial or lateral area of the tendo achillis respectively and taken towards the plantar surface of the foot.

PLANTAR SURFACE. Long strokes are placed from the heel to the metatarsophalangeal joints, steadying the foot by placing the other hand on the dorsum in a similar manner to the hand treatment. The medial and lateral borders of the plantar surface should be treated particularly well as the plantar vessels pass along these borders. It is essential to apply the strokes very firmly in order to avoid any tickling sensation. In the very rare cases where treatment is necessary the toes are treated on their plantar surface in the same way as described for the fingers. Where a tickling sensation occurs the plantar surface should be treated along the medial and lateral border with short strokes, placed at right angles to the surface of the foot, passing from the lateral or medial aspect of the foot towards the plantar surface.

Anterior aspect of trunk

The strokes described in this section serve two purposes. In early treatment sessions, when spontaneous increased tissue tension (which is very often relieved during the treatment of the dorsal regions of the trunk) appears anteriorly, the strokes in the region of the iliac crest and subcostal margins should be used as routine strokes. In later treatment sessions it will be possible to carry the iliac crest strokes and the subcostal strokes forward in the normal sitting position used for treatment wherever possible. In these patients it will therefore not be necessary to terminate the treatment in the lying position. In some conditions (*e.g.*, menstrual disturbances) these strokes will constitute part of the specific treatment and will therefore have to be continued and applied in every treatment session. The strokes described in this section over the rest of the anterior chest wall should never be applied as routine treatment. They sometimes represent an additional help in specific conditions (*e.g.*, asthma) when the dorsal areas of the same segments show improvement in tension. The strokes over the anterior aspect of the pelvic region are mentioned by the German originator of this method as helpful in menstrual and uterine disturbances.

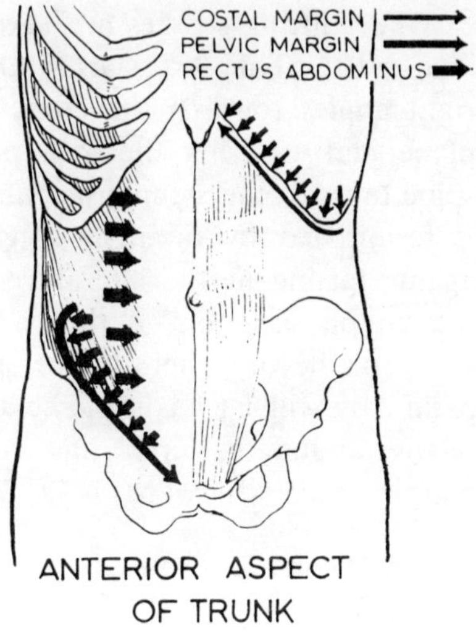

FIG. 39

Subcostal margin

Short lifting strokes are taken at short intervals along the costal margin. They are started above the margin and directed at right angles towards the margin, starting at the lateral vertical plane and covering the area towards the xiphoid process. The treatment of this area is terminated by taking a long stroke along the subcostal margin, again starting at the lateral vertical plane and continuing towards the end of the sternum, if this is possible. Should the fingers be stopped by the resistance of the tissue, the stroke is terminated at the lateral border of rectus abdominis. A curious sensation of skin irritation will be experienced by most patients over the medial condyle of the humerus on the homolateral side when the finger passes over the junction of the 7th to the 8th rib (Fig. 39).

Pelvic margin

Short lifting strokes are taken at short intervals along the iliac crest. They are started above the crest and directed at right angles towards the crest, starting at the lateral vertical plane and covering the area past the anterior superior iliac spine towards the symphysis pubis. The treatment of this area is terminated by taking a long stroke just above the crest, again starting at the lateral vertical plane and continuing to the symphysis pubis, if this is possible. Should the cutting sensation beyond the anterior superior iliac spine become too painful it will be advisable to treat the lateral margin of the rectus abdominis first, and return to the complete pelvic margin stroke afterwards (Fig. 39).

Rectus abdominis

The lateral margin of the rectus abdominis is treated in a manner similar to the technique applied to the margin of latissimus dorsi. Short lifting strokes are applied at right angles to the margin of the muscles. It is advisable to ascertain the position of the rectus sheath by asking the patient to lift the head against a resistance applied by the hand to the forehead.

Anterior chest region

The German originator of C.T.M. mentions the strokes described under this heading as helpful in cases of resistant asthma where other therapeutic measures, such as relaxation and breathing exercises alone, have not proved fully successful. The author has tried this treatment on one patient with very resistant asthma and it proved very helpful. It is essential to treat the back, including the basic section, simultaneously. The anterior chest region should not be treated unless it has been preceded by four to six treatment sessions of the whole back. Prior to the treatment of the chest region the tension in the lower abdominal region should be relieved. The patient is treated in the lying position with a small supporting pillow under the thighs to relieve the tension on the abdominal muscles. Small lifting strokes are directed towards the sternum in the intercostal spaces. These are followed by treatment of the subcostal margin. If the patient is not distressed the treatment of the thoracic inlet follows. Small strokes are directed towards the sternoclavicular articulation and along the interclavicular ligament. Transverse strokes across the region of the angle of Ludwig terminate the treatment of this area which must be followed again by treatment of the subcostal margin.

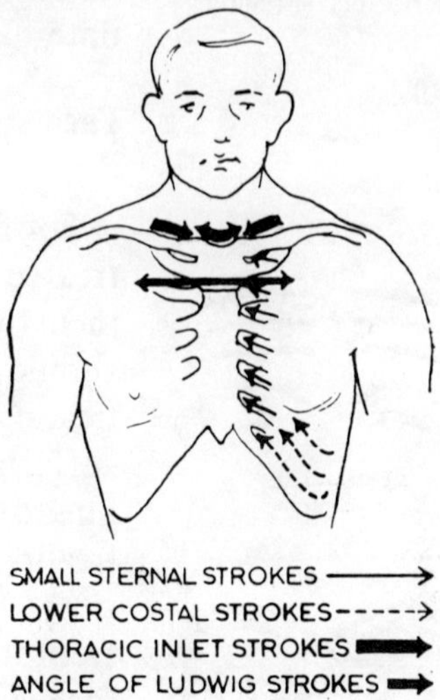

FIG. 40
Anterior chest region.

Anterior pelvic region

C.T.M. in this region is reported to be helpful in patients with menstrual disturbances or uterine dysfunction. Treatment of the sacral region must precede the stimulation of the anterior

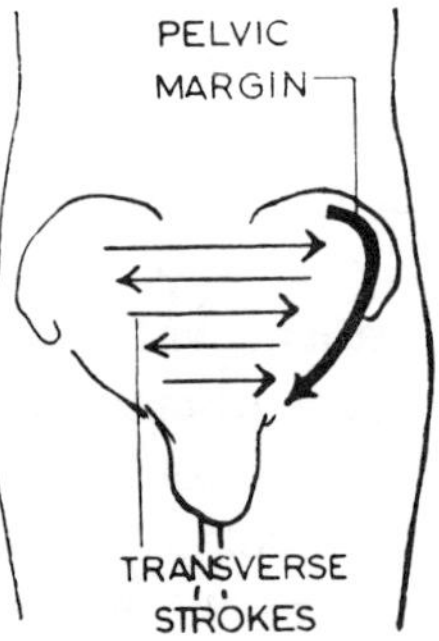

FIG. 41
Anterior pelvic region.

aspect. For the strokes described under this heading the patient is in the lying or the crook lying position. The pelvic margin is first treated with a stroke starting above the iliac crest, past the anterior superior iliac spine towards the symphysis pubis. This is followed by transverse strokes across the pelvic inlet, starting at the hair border and progressing in a cranial direction as far as the level of the anterior superior iliac spines. These strokes are carried out with alternate hands.

Face

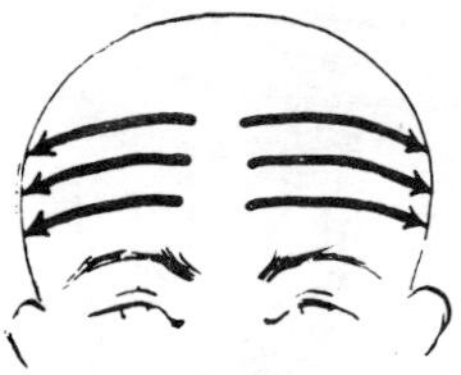

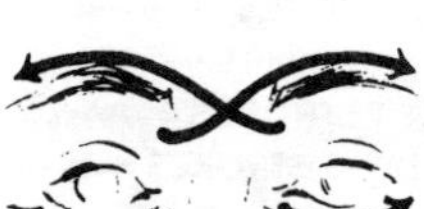

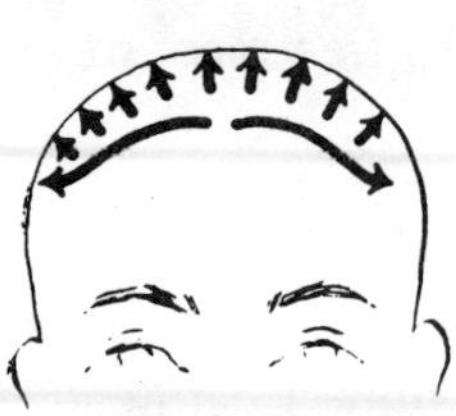

For facial treatment the patient is best treated in the lying position. This treatment will not often be necessary, but should never be attempted without first treating the whole back. In most patients suffering from headaches relief will already have been obtained when treating the scapular and cervical regions in the back. In a few patients suffering from frontal headaches, treatment of the face will prove beneficial. Chronic sinusitis is a condition which sometimes responds beneficially to facial treatment in addition to treatment of the back.

To start the treatment, strokes are applied bimanually from the midline of the face towards the temporal region. It is advisable to hold the fingers at a fairly acute angle so that the strokes are not too deep. Short lifting strokes are then applied along the border of occipitofron-

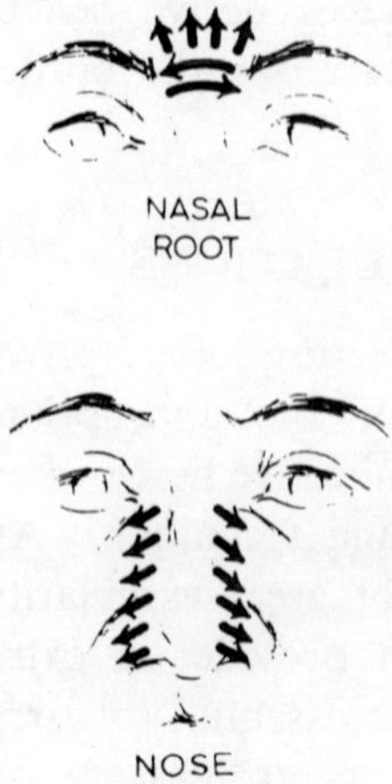

Fig. 42
Anterior aspect of face.

talis, terminating the treatment of this area again with bimanually applied long strokes from midline towards the temporal region. A bimanually applied stroke is then taken above the orbit, starting the stroke by crossing the hands in the midline. The inferior border of the orbit is treated with a single stroke starting at the lateral border of the nose and giving slight countertraction to the skin with the other hand. The nasal area is treated with short strokes passing from one medial angle of the eye across the root of the nose to the medial angle of the other eye. When necessary, because of nasal congestion, short strokes are taken simultaneously with both hands, starting at the nasal septum and stroking towards the lateral border of the nose. The treatment is terminated by applying flat-handed effleurage strokes from the midline towards the lateral border of the face.

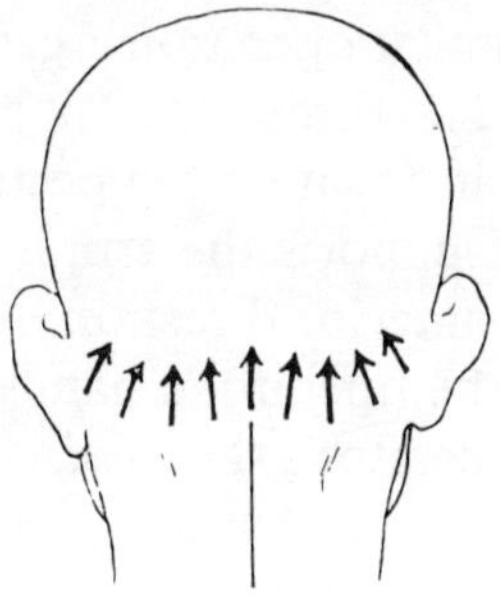

POSTERIOR ASPECT OF HEAD
Fig. 43

Posterior aspect of head

Patients suffering from occipital headaches derive benefit from the application of short lifting strokes along the border of attachment of occipitofrontalis at the back.

SPECIAL STRETCHING MANIPULATIONS

The manipulations described in this section often prove useful when terminating the treatment of the appropriate area. They provide a final stretch on the connective tissue when tension has already been relieved by stroking technique. All these manipulations take place in regions of great vascularity and in the author's experience very often provide an extra stimulus to the peripheral circulation. It is essential to carry them out with great care in order not to exert pressure on superficially placed nervous structures.

Axilla

The operator stands on the homolateral side of the axilla under treatment. For the right axilla the ulnar three fingers of the right hand are placed against the latissimus dorsi fascia, while the left hand supports the patient's arm in abduction. Traction is now applied in a posterior direction on the posterior wall of the axilla. A similar operation is carried out on the fascia of pectoralis major. The three ulnar fingers of the operator's left hand are placed in front of the pectoralis major tendon, while the right hand supports the arm in abduction. Traction is now applied in an anterior direction. A final stretch can be applied by crossing the operator's hands and supporting the patient's arm on the operator's shoulder. A simultaneous stretch is then carried out by both hands against the posterior and anterior wall of the axilla (Figs. 44, 45, 46).

Elbow

The operator stands slightly behind the patient on the homolateral side, placing the posterior aspect of the elbow joint into the combined palms of both hands. The fingers come to lie anteriorly across the joint. The hands move simultaneously, each hand moving away from the midline, thus providing a stretch on the anterior covering of the antecubital fossa (Fig. 47).

Palm

A transverse stretch can be applied to the palmar fascia by placing the fingers of the operator's two hands across the patient's palm, both thumbs being placed above the hand. The stretch is applied by moving the fingers of the operator's hands simultaneously away from the midline (Fig. 48).

Foot

A manipulation similar to that used for the hand can be applied to provide stretch for the plantar fascia, the operator's thumbs resting against the dorsum of the foot.

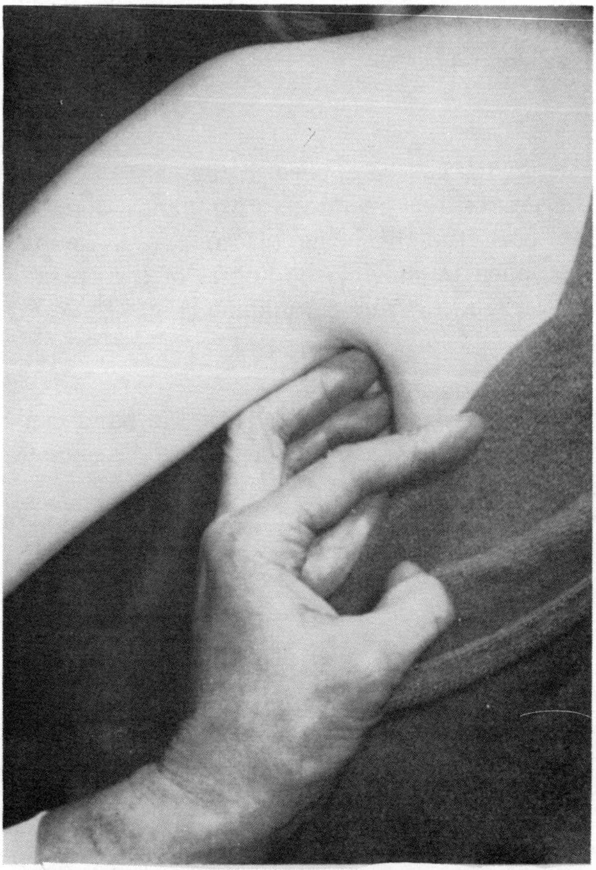

Fig. 44

Stretching manipulations.

Stretching of posterior axillary wall.

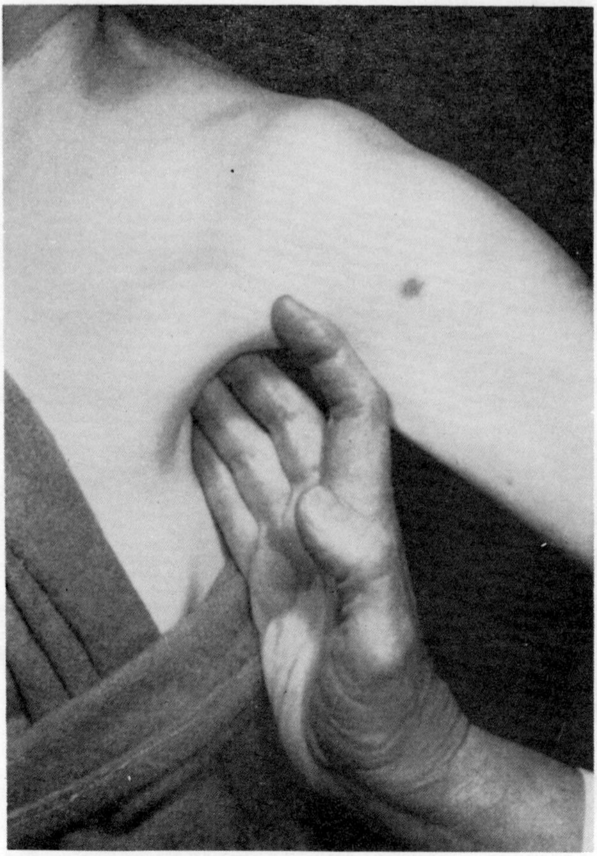

Fig. 45
Stretching manipulations.
Stretching of anterior axillary wall.

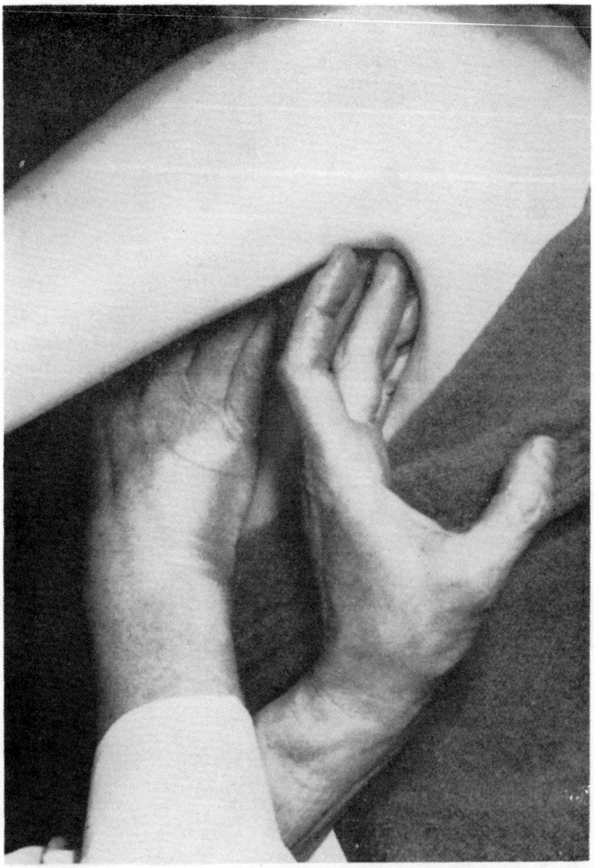

FIG. 46

Stretching manipulations.

Bimanual stretch of axilla.

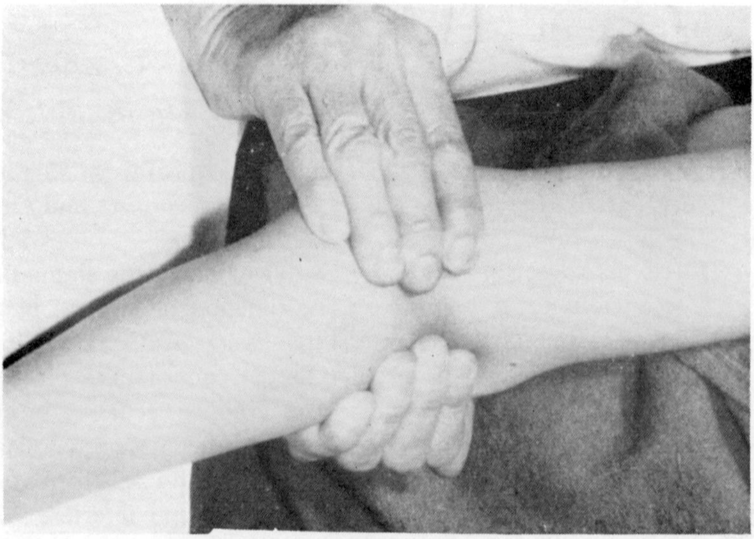

Fig. 47
Stretching manipulations.
Stretching of antecubital fossa.

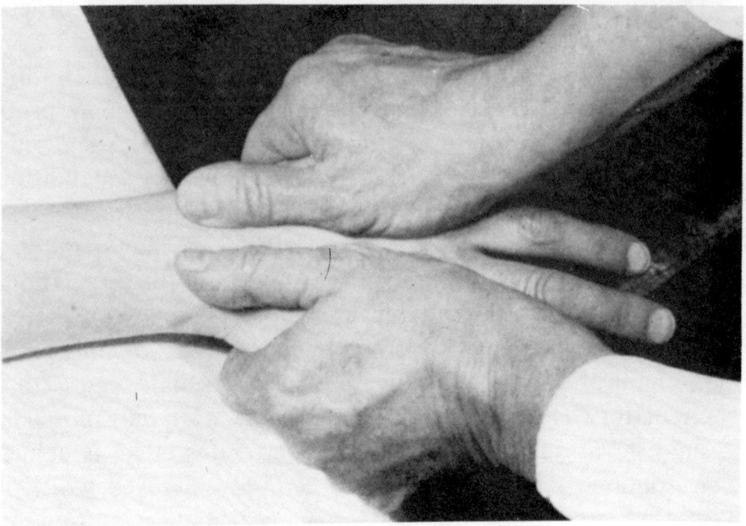

Fig. 48
Stretching manipulations.
Palmar stretch.

CHAPTER VII

Effect of Connective Tissue Manipulation

Hippocrates: All parts of The Human Organism form a circle. Every part is therefore at the same time *Beginning* and *End.*

THE massage will eventually always influence the circulation to various types of tissue. The function of viscera, blood vessels, supporting tissue (interstitial tissue) or tissue destined to produce movement (muscular tissue) cannot take place in an isolated manner. Pathological conditions occurring in any one structure must eventually reflect on other tissues. Inflammation in a viscus, spasm in vascular walls, and scar formation in any tissue must have widespread effects and interfere with the function of the whole organism, as all structures function interdependently. It is impossible to visualize changes in skin texture without realizing that cutaneous circulatory changes must affect also the circulation to muscles, organs and nerves. The pathological changes may originate in deep-lying structures and eventually become apparent in superficial tissues as discovered by Head (1898) and by Mackenzie (1917). Interference with superficial circulation by scar tissue may produce pathological conditions in distant parts of the body, as discussed by Nonnenbruch and Gross (1952). Reactive adaptation is therefore possible in both directions. It may pass from deeper lying structures to the body surface or it may pass in the opposite direction. The massage influences the circulation on the body surface in selected areas and so opens up increased circulatory pathways to other regions of the organism. The mechanical tension stimulus is the immediate cause of the circulatory effect. At the present time it is only possible to suggest various explanations as to how this effect is achieved. Autonomic reflex pathways are certainly involved which may also be responsible for endocrine participation in the result. More and more evidence appears of the importance which mast cells play in alterations in the ground substance of connective tissue. Heparin and histamine, which are present in the granules of the cell, are released by appropriate stimulation. It is therefore impossible to discard the possibility of participation of these cells in the effect of the massage. The terminal vascular reticulum is stimulated directly by the massage stroke. Its widespread connections explain the diffuse and widespread effect of the massage. The effects will therefore be local at or near the area of stimulation and general affecting the whole organism.

The type of reaction will always be the same. Its intensity and duration may vary, depending on the severity of the pathological condition and the strength of the stimulus.

It will be convenient to consider the reactions under three headings:—

1. Sensation of the patient.
2. Skin reaction.
3. General reaction.

Sensation of the patient

When the tensile stroke is applied to healthy tissue, the patient will report a very slight scratching or cutting sensation. Applying the stroke to tissues with increased tension will produce a *very sharp* cutting sensation which is obtained with application of very little pressure and a very decreased angle of impact of the fingers on the skin. This sharp cutting or scratching sensation is typical of the correct application of technique. It is also indicative of a satisfactory circulatory response. As tension decreases, so the intensity of the cutting sensation decreases. Under certain conditions the patient may report a sensation of deep, dull pressure, which shows no relation to the pressure actually applied by the finger. This feeling of dull pressure often becomes apparent when passing through areas of elevation or swelling. It may also occur while working in the upper areas of the back. This sensation is an indication that tension is unrelieved in lower segments, *i.e.* segments nearer the sacral areas, or that a circulatory reaction is not obtained. By returning to the lower segments a sensation of severe cutting is often experienced by the patient. As soon as the caudal sections have become normalized, a return to the upper sections will show that the sensations have now changed. The sensation of pressure has given way to a cutting sensation, showing that the tension in these areas has become more superficial. It is the author's belief that the sensation of dull pressure is due to deep congestion which, under the influence of the massage, is increased because more distant channels are not yet open. A very similar sensation is often reported by patients under application of (ultra-short wave) diathermy to the trapezius region for paraesthesia of the upper limbs. The cutting sensation cannot be produced with any other type of massage. It is an indication of the satisfactory progress of the treatment. To continue in areas of pressure does not achieve any beneficial results. Sometimes patients may report that the sensation becomes unbearable. It is possible to decrease the cutting sensation by decreasing the speed of the stroke. Increase in speed increases the cutting in abnormally tense tissue. The speed of the stroke must therefore be adapted to the resistance experienced when stroking through the tissues. Sometimes patients are not very definite in their report about the type of sensation experienced. In these cases it is advisable to confine the massage to areas where a clear cutting sensation can be obtained. Sometimes patients report a more or less intense tickling sensation when the stroke is applied. This indicates an unsatisfactory circulatory response. The tickling often appears during the application of long strokes over the iliac crest or the subcostal area. It may be changed by short lifting strokes at right angles to the direction of the previously applied long stroke or by treating caudally situated areas. It may be changed sometimes by applying stimulating strokes to two trigger points in the sacral area. One such point is the trigonum lumborum where fascial contact can easily be established between the muscular gap of abdominus externus and latissimus dorsi. A short sharp stroke is passed in the triangle vertically down towards the iliac crest. The posterior aspect of the great trochanter of the femur is another point of stimulation. It may be very difficult to obtain the correct sensory response in the presence of conditions showing vascular spasm. In these cases treatment should be confined to the sacral and buttock

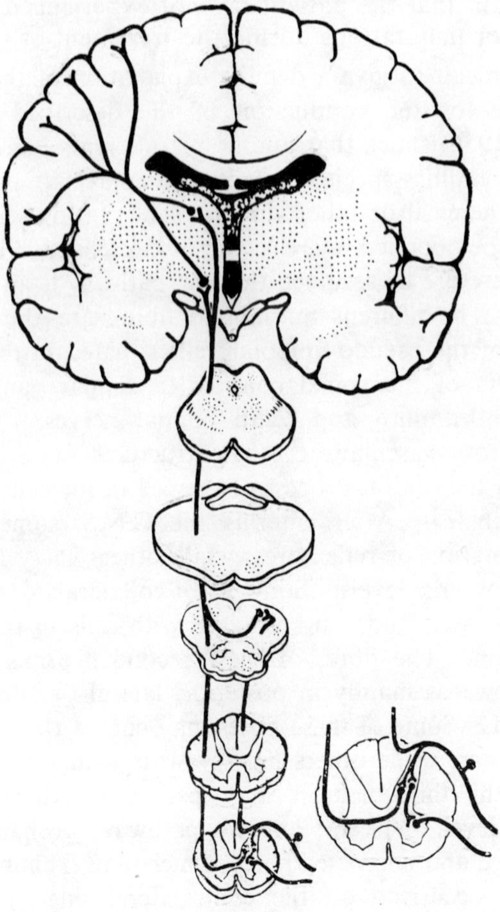

FIG. 49
Diagram showing probable route of ascending (afferent) autonomic pathways from the cord to the brain. (Mitchell: *Cardiovascular Innervation.*)

areas until a response can be obtained. Careful attention to technique will usually be successful after a few treatment sessions. Should this prove impossible, it must be assumed that vascular changes have become irreversible. Before terminating any treatment session the operator must ascertain that the patient has no longer any sensations present in the treated areas apart from warmth. Careful questioning must also make certain that the patient has not experienced headache, dyspnoea or palpitations during the treatment or afterwards.

It is difficult to give a definite explanation of the pathways responsible for the conduction of the described sensations. Mitchell (1956) states that autonomic afferents convey impressions from endings specially adapted to appreciate pain, stretch, pressure, chemical or other stimuli. The cutting sensation can frequently be obtained in areas where skin sensation is impaired. It must therefore be assumed that the pathway is an autonomic pathway. The afferent autonomic fibres are the peripheral processes of the pseudo-unipolar cells situated in the posterior root ganglia of the spinal cord or in similar ganglia of the fifth, seventh, ninth and tenth cranial nerves. They carry impulses from vascular or other structures under autonomic control via the central process of the cell to the central nervous system (C.N.S.). After entering the C.N.S. some take part in the formation of reflex arcs, while others carry impulses to higher autonomic levels. Some axon collaterals pass vertically and transversely, and some synapse with cells in the posterior grey column. The fibres of these second neurons may cross or pass upwards mainly in posterior, lateral or anterior tracts of the cord. Some of these fibres may end in the thalamus or hypothalamus, while others may synapse with new cells. The fibres of the third neuron may pass to cortical and thus conscious level. Visceral afferent pathways probably contain both crossed and uncrossed fibres, which may explain sensations sometimes occurring on the contralateral side of the body. Figure 49 may help to illustrate this explanation.

Skin reaction

On applying the tensile stroke to healthy skin a two-fold reaction can be observed. The first reaction to appear is a red line confined to the area of the stroke. It appears a few seconds after the stroke has been applied, reaches its height in 30 to 60 seconds, and fades very gradually. It may have disappeared in a few minutes or it may last for more than an hour. The intensity of this red band and the duration of its existence are influenced by the strength of the stimulus and by the number of times this stimulus is repeated. Both factors increase the intensity and duration of the reaction. When the stroke stimulus is strong or repeated several times over the same line, a second visible reaction can be observed. The reddening is no longer confined to the line of the stroke, but spreads beyond it after a further delay of a few seconds. Beyond the line of the original stroke a red flush develops which may spread for a varying distance. The outline of the flush or flare is not well defined and starts to fade sooner than the original stroke line. The more intense the colour of this flare, the longer the time taken for its disappearance. On sensitive skin or by repeating the stroke several times with sufficient intensity, a third reaction can be observed. Along the line of the original stroke and often slightly beyond it, a slight swelling appears which is surrounded by the flare. This swelling is termed a "wheal" and may take up to three minutes to appear. It gradually becomes paler and loses its well-defined outline, but it may take hours to disappear. The above reactions to a stroke stimulus constitute the *triple response* as discussed by Lewis (1927). (Niebauer, 1972). The first reaction is always present; the other two depend on the strength of the stimulus and the number of its repetitions.

In applying the C.T.M. stroke the skin reaction always follows the above described sequence of events. The intensity of the reaction depends on the initial tension present in the tissue under treatment, the depth of the stroke applied, the speed of the movement, and the number of repetitions of the stroke over the same area. Repeating the stroke more than nine or ten times does not seem to increase the reaction. A repetition of three is essential. The duration of the reaction also depends on the initial tension present in the tissue. It is possible to observe the presence of the skin reaction after twenty-four hours or longer. The fading time of the skin reaction decreases as tissue tension decreases. At the end of a treatment session on skin with no pathological tension, both skin and cutting reactions are very slight and the skin reaction disappears after a few minutes.

Bruising as a Skin Reaction. Some patients, especially rheumatoid patients who bruise very easily, may after several hours show small subcutaneous bruises. These are not painful and usually only appear after the first two to four treatments. The pathological tissue changes associated with rheumatic diseases probably include an abnormal permeability of subcutaneous tissue which gradually disappears as the condition improves. If these bruises are painful, the technique may be at fault. The appearance of these bruises is no contraindication to the massage treatment. It might however be advisable to warn the patient and reassure her.

Circulatory disturbances due to vascular spasm form an exception to the previously described sequence of events resulting in the triple response. At first it is only possible to obtain a faint stroke reaction after repeated application of the stroke without any flare or wheal. In all cases of satisfactory progress of the treatment, the response improves with each treatment until it is possible to obtain a wheal. From that point the treatment follows the usual pattern, *i.e.* the response becomes less violent. The improvement in peripheral circulation coincides with a less violent reaction in response to the massage stroke.

Summary of Skin Reactions. Following the massage stroke a well-defined red line appears confined to the area of the stroke. This reaction appears in skin areas which have lost their sensory innervation. It must therefore be assumed that it is due to a dilatation of minute vessels and is independent of the somatic supply of the skin area. It is possible that the terminal reticulum of the capillaries is stimulated by the stroke but it seems impossible that the dilatation is due to a nervous reflex which is dependent on somatic innervation.

The author has only been able to obtain the flare reaction in skin with intact sensory supply. According to Lewis (1927) the flare is due to a widespread dilatation of skin arterioles which is brought about through the axon reflex. The reflex starts in a somatic sensory fibre of the skin, passes centrally as far as the next division of this fibre and causes an efferent impulse to pass peripherally along a collateral of the same fibre which ends in the coat of an arteriole. This results in a vaso-dilatation of the supplied vessel.

The third part of the response is the wheal which appears over the original primary stroke line. According to Lewis (1927) the wheal is due to increased permeability of the vessel wall. This can be proved by testing the protein contents of the wheal fluid which is almost identical with the protein contents of serum and greater than the protein contents of lymph collected from the part. As the wheal only appears in response to a strong stimulus which is the result of increased tissue tension, it must be assumed that it will be associated with injury to some tissue cells. The substance liberated in response to the cell injury is considered by Lewis (1927) to be a histamine-related substance. Further research may reveal that the mast cells of the connective tissue element of the skin are associated with the liberation of a histamine-related substance. The work of Professor Niebauer and al. has established the presence of cell structures which change function under pathological conditions. This may help in the future to obtain a better understanding of the reactions after application of C.T.M. and also open the use of it in a wider field of pathological conditions.

General reactions

The information given in previous chapters about the close relations of somatic and autonomic nervous systems will make it understandable that alterations of a pathological as well as a physiological nature must cause repercussions not only in the close vicinity of the stimulus but eventually in distant parts of the organism. Pathological alterations on the body surface due to distant foci have been described by Head (1898), Mackenzie (1917) and Dicke (1953). Connective tissue massage attempts to influence the pathological alterations on the body surface as far as these can be influenced by alterations in the circulation. The circulation on the body surface is however not an isolated network of blood vessels. These vessels only represent the terminal branches of the blood vascular tree, which carries the fluid to bathe *all* cellular elements of the organism. Barcroft and Swan (1953) have experimentally established the existence of peripheral vasodilator nerve fibres. Chemical vasodilator substances may also prove to be responsible for the peripheral vasodilatation. The existence of an increased peripheral circulation due to the massage manipulations must be considered an established fact. Völker and Rostovsky (1949) have carried out experimental measurements and proved that the skin temperature increased after application of the massage, reaching its maximum approximately half-an-hour after termination of the massage. Dr Woodmansey and the author carried out investigations on a small number of patients in 1957 and could record increases of skin temperature of the foot in three patients varying from 1° to 2° C. In all the investigated patients the massage was only carried out for approximately twenty minutes in the sacral and lumbar segments of the back. A single experiment carried out by the author at a Viennese clinic, measuring blood flow in the lower extremity, proved increase in blood flow, reaching its maximum seventeen minutes after termination of the massage, which again had only been applied to the back.

The German originators of the massage claim an increase of sweat production in many patients after application of the massage. The experiments of Woodmansey and Ebner attempted to measure skin resistance due to increase of skin moisture in the hands during application of the massage. In all the patients the skin resistance decreased. One patient reported profuse sweating for several days. It is quite clear that many more scientific investigations will have to be carried out to establish the exact mode of action of the various phenomena resulting from the massage application. The clinical experiences and the results of the few experimental attempts however make it clear that the massage has far-reaching effects, not only influencing the peripheral circulation but effecting general constitutional changes and influencing the function of the viscera. Visceral temperature changes, which necessarily must affect the blood supply of the organ due to changes in peripheral segmental temperature changes, have been reported in the literature (Best and Taylor, 1961). These effects must take place via nervous pathways as they can be observed distant from the area of application and some must take place as humoral reactions as they can be observed a considerable time after termination of the massage. Some of these effects will be discussed below. It is very important to be aware of them as they may be either beneficial or detrimental to the patient.

PERSPIRATION. Some patients start to perspire profusely during the treatment, and sometimes continue for a considerable time after termination of the treatment. This does not apply only to patients who are inclined to perspire freely on the slightest provocation; but it is especially applicable to patients who usually do not perspire or only with difficulty. According to Teirich-Leube (1960) this type of perspiration is due to parasympathetic stimulation.

CHANGE IN PERIPHERAL TEMPERATURE. Patients often report spontaneously that the extremities, such as the hands or feet, feel warm. This occurs during treatment of the back without local application in the periphery. In the author's experience this amazing result was obtained in patients with flail limbs after A.P.M., and might serve to illustrate the fact that the vascular innervation is very irregular and the appropriate nerve cells might be situated anywhere in the course of the vessels.

RELIEF OF VISCERAL FUNCTIONAL SYMPTOMS. Patients suffering from dyspnoea, *e.g.* following frequent asthma attacks, suddenly report that they can breathe freely and deeply.

RELIEF OF VISCERAL PAIN. Patients with gastric discomfort without pathological stomach changes suddenly report that the stomach pain has completely disappeared.

German authors (Teirich-Leube, 1960) report that as a result of the massage the general basic state of the autonomic system becomes slightly emphasized on the parasympathetic side. In the author's experience patients who were depressed because they felt unable to cope with the various demands of their professional or domestic life, became cheerful, slept better and

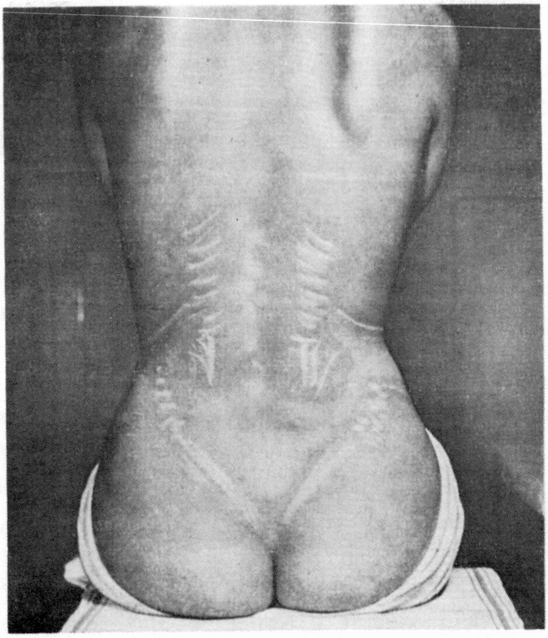

FIG. 50
Back showing (*a*) red line, (*b*) flush, (*c*) wheal.

regained a sense of proportion towards the important and not so important factors in their life. Patients often report a general feeling of well-being. In some patients a feeling of general fatigue appears one to two hours after termination of treatment. which allows them to go to sleep easily.

The overall effect of the massage seems to be improvement of circulation to all structures including supporting tissues. muscle and nerves. It thereby helps to restore the balance between the two parts of the autonomic system. It is essential to observe carefully the patient's reaction and attempt to obtain an overall balance and not only a shifting of symptoms. Due to the continuity of connective tissue throughout the body it is possible to relieve existing tension in one part by allowing it to appear somewhere else. Experience will soon make the operator conversant with some of the danger signals but it may prove useful to mention the more frequent mistakes.

EXCESSIVE TREATMENT. It must be realised that an extensive peripheral vasodilatation may produce a condition similar to shock. It may lower the blood pressure in specially sensitive individuals, and cause a feeling of depression, headache and general malaise.

VISCERAL SYMPTOMS IN AUTONOMICALLY LABILE PATIENTS. In order to avoid symptoms such as palpitations or dyspnoea, it is advisable to observe the patient carefully while treating the appropriate dermatomes in the back. When applying stimulating strokes to preganglionic fibres, *i.e.* short strokes on either side of the thoracic spine, it is essential to intersperse the treatment with strokes stimulating postganglionic fibres, *e.g.* strokes to the anterior aspect of the chest and particularly the subcostal region.

HEADACHE. Headache or a sensation of nausea sometimes appears during the treatment of shoulder and cervical segments. This may be due to the stimulation of vagal fibres, and can easily be relieved by applying strokes on the anterior aspect of these areas, *i.e.* over the forehead and upper chest areas.

TRANSFERENCE OF TENSION. Treatment of areas of increased tension in the back may sometimes result in the sudden appearance of tension areas on the anterior aspect of the body. This applies particularly to the shoulder and cervical region where the sternomastoid may suddenly appear contracted. These symptoms can easily be relieved by treatment of the anterior aspect.

CIRCULATORY DISTURBANCES. When treating dorsal segments, paraesthesia may suddenly appear in the appropriate extremities in the form of a " pins and needles " sensation. In the upper limb intensive treatment of the axillary and latissimus dorsi areas, and in the lower limb treatment of the great trochanter and iliotibial tract areas, rapidly relieves the symptoms.

To summarize the effect of C.T.M., provided the stimulus given has been adequate and correctly applied:

General effect

It will help to harmonize the relationship between the *Sympathetic* and *Parasympathetic* part of the *Autonomic Nervous System* by increasing the blood supply to parasympathetic nuclei in the pelvic region.

WITHIN THE SEGMENT. It will help to normalize the circulation between organs and organ-systems and other tissues belonging to the same segment or number of segments.

LOCALLY. It will improve the bloodsupply of the surface tissues in the area under treatment in particular the Connective Tissue Element in tissues such as muscle.

STIMULUS STRENGTH.

Too weak a stimulus – no result.
Adequate stimulus – harmonizing
Too strong a stimulus – emphasizes over reaction of sympathetic side of Autonomic System (Intensive pain calls up Defence Reaction–sympathetic and suprarenal stimulation).

Finally it must be remembered that no structure in the Human Organism can function in an isolated manner and no stimulus applied anywhere can remain isolated.

GENERAL RULES. The patient should have no sensation

apart from warmth after termination of the massage. Any sensation still present, such as a memory of the stroke sensation in the tissues, must be removed before the patient is permitted to go home. Usually all peripheral sensations can be easily removed by treating the great trochanter area and/or the subcostal areas.

Sometimes more serious disturbances occur in patients with a very labile Autonomic Nervous System. These may be: Headaches–Palpitations–a feeling of general collapse. These patients should immediately be made to lye down, first in side–lying to treat the sacral area–then in back–lying to treat peripherally the Great Trochanter Area and the Ilio-Tibial Tract–if necessary anterior pelvic and sub-costal areas. The patient will *not* suffer lasting damage but can feel very uncomfortable if *Basic Rules* are not observed. For the clinical worker the following summary of incorrect reactions may prove useful.

Bruising as a Skin Reaction

This is not a contra-indication to continue with the treatment. The bruise is only superficial and painless. In these patients the bruising no longer occurs after 2-4 treatments and was due to a temporary presence of fragility of superficial small vessels. If the bruise is painful the technique of the stroke should be revised.

Lack of correct cutting sensation

1) No sensation obtained after application of 3-10 repetitive strokes
   a) revise accuracy of technique
   b) return to more caudally situated areas
   c) stimulate circulatory Trigger points
      These are:
      In the Pelvis: Trigonum Lumborum
      around Greater Trochanter
      Point medial to Ischial
      Tuberosity

In the Leg:

- Adductor Hiatus
- Soleal Arch

In the Upper Limb:

- Axilla
- Inferior scapular angle

All these are points where circulatory channels become fairly superficial and an attempt is made to stimulate the nerve endings in the vessels.

A very important factor concerning technique is the pain sensation during the stroke. The cutting sensation must never be painful to the patient, it must always be acceptable. This must be explained to the patient, who sometimes considers that the more painful the treatment, the more successful it will be. "Pain" calls up the defence mechanism of the body which includes peripheral vaso-constriction which defeats the aim of the treatment. The stroke must therefore be reduced in depth or speed or changed from long to short stroke.

CHAPTER VIII

Therapeutic Application

General considerations

In the following chapters an attempt is made to give some information about the application of connective tissue massage (C.T.M.) in pathological conditions. It is hoped that future experience and a more universal application of this method may provide further valuable insight into the pathology and therapy of a number of conditions. It would be a grave mistake to discard valuable therapeutic agents which are giving satisfactory results. There are, however, many pathological conditions where medical applications or medical and physiotherapeutic applications combined do not succeed in restoring the health of the patient, and in a number of cases do not even succeed in alleviating the symptoms which prevent the patient from leading a satisfactory and useful life. The experience of the German originator, the information given by many German practitioners, both doctors and physiotherapists, and the experience of the author and her colleagues are convincing proof that C.T.M. may represent a very valuable additional therapeutic agent if correctly applied. The physician or surgeon will refer the patient, with a well-founded diagnosis, to a trained physiotherapist for treatment. The physiotherapist is specially trained to observe tissue changes (both visually and manually), initial changes and changes resulting from the application of special massage techniques. The additional information usually readily supplied by the patient to the physiotherapist should enable her/him to become a valued collaborator of the doctor. It is hoped that the information given in this book will help to achieve this, not by displacing old proved therapeutic agents, but by adding a new one. Medical research in the last decade has proved that the conception of an isolated pathological process anywhere in the human body can no longer be maintained.

The abnormal functioning of any organ or tissue in the body will invariably influence the functioning of the whole organism. Connective tissue massage may be one of the agents which may help to harmonize the disturbed function by activating nervous, hormonal and humoral pathways.

The science of *Physiology* teaches us the normal function of The Human Organism—the science of *Pathology* teaches the deviations from the normal and the science of *Therapeutics* should teach us what can be done to make changes retrograde provided they have not become irreversible. *Universal Function* of the organism as a whole must depend on restoration of *universal vascular interchange*—if this is impossible an attempt must be made to restore this interchange as far as possible.

C.T.M. is a unique help in this attempt. It is essential to sort out the various therapeutic agents—consider their effect and use them logically on a sound scientific basis. At present it is impossible to explain in all instances empirically beneficial effects. This applies to Drug-therapy as well as Physiotherapy. New pathological, anatomical and physiological discoveries will continue to explain some of these empirical effects but we must never forget that brain *and* hand must continue to work together. One criterion however must not be violated. No therapeutic approach must ever be detrimental to the patient. This certainly can be said of C.T.M. and has been proved during the past thirty years.

From a treatment point of view two main groups of conditions will be considered:

1. Changes in peripheral structures due to interference with their blood supply. In some cases the cause for the dysfunction will be known; in a number of cases it will be only partly understood in the light of present day knowledge.

2. Changes in peripheral structures which have occurred due to pathological conditions existing or having existed in other parts of the segmental distribution.

In all cases the body must be considered as a whole and no attempt should be made to start the treatment by concentrating in the first few treatments on the areas of maximal symptomatic disturbance.

Every treatment must therefore start in the sacral area and in most cases should not progress beyond the basic section until a clear cutting or scratching sensation is obtained in that area. Exceptions to this rule will be discussed under individual treatments.

Before describing individual treatments, it might be useful to summarize some of the factors discussed in greater detail in previous chapters.

The influence of manual traction applied to blood vessels is very small. The amount of traction applied with the C.T.M. stroke will therefore only have to be considered in order to concentrate the main effect on the cutaneous, subcutaneous or fascial layer of the body surface. This depth of the stroke can be altered by changing the angle of the stroking finger in relation to the surface under treatment. It must be stressed that skin friction must always be avoided as it affects only the epidermis which is almost avascular. The immediate response to the stroke will affect the superficial capillary field by the mechanical tensile stimulus which results in nervous, hormonal and humeral responses. It might also be considered important that comparatively large venous vessels depend on patent vasa vasorum as the vein itself carries deoxygenated blood, and the latter can therefore contribute very little to metabolic functioning of the cells of the vessel wall. Stagnation in the venous part of the circulation is responsible for a vicious circle because it results in oedema in the tissue spaces which causes collapse of lymph capillaries. This will impede the return of colloid substances and so increase the osmotic pressure of tissue spaces. Dilatation and increase of permeability of blood capillaries achieved by the C.T.M. stroke will facilitate colloid return.

The arterioles deep to the subpapillary plexuses show strong muscular coats and are therefore probably more readily influenced by nervous stimuli. The importance of the cutting sensation which must pass via nervous pathways may be explained as proof that the tensile stimulus has reached the deeper arterial plexuses. The distant sensory irritation sometimes following the stroke may be caused by the fact that the stimulus follows vascular and not somatic afferents.

Records

It is essential to investigate every patient very carefully, and note the findings on a back chart before the first treatment. These investigations must be carried out with an absolutely open mind and not with the intention of finding some alterations. It is essential to note carefully at each session the area which has been treated. Any report from the patient about his condition in the interval between treatments must be recorded as well as any changes observed during treatment. This permits the treatment to be adapted to varying conditions and gives a picture of the progress and improvement of the patient. As previously stressed, questions addressed to the patient must be in no way suggestive, but it is important to give a short explanation to the patient in order to obtain his co-operation which is essential. All this may take a little time, but it should be considered time well spent. No patient should be on treatment for years as sometimes happens with some forms of physiotherapy. If no results are obtained within two weeks the whole situation should be reconsidered and reported to the doctor.

A short outline of treatment procedure may prove helpful in planning the treatment.

1st Treatment:

Name – Age – Occupation – Medical Diagnosis – if possible B.P.

History of Patient's complaint–primarily – *Pain – Functional Disability*

Back Inspection and record

Treatment: Usually only Basic Section–sometimes progressing into thigh or towards axilla–Latissimus Dorsi.

2nd Treatment: if possible the following day

Enquiry about result of previous treatment: Pain – Function – Bruises.

General Condition: Sleep,–,fatigue – appetite – bowel function.

Treatment: Modify treatment resulting from report of patient (satisfactory repeat previous treatment), tired–give rest before allowed to go home, restless–less deep and aim for less sharp reaction etc.

3rd Treatment: if possible again the following day

By now one should have a picture of the patient's reaction.

Progression: If the reaction is satisfactory, progress further up the back into the arm–down the leg–reach as soon as possible the area primarily affected.

Interval: At first 3 times per week–improvement–progress to twice a week–to once a week–once a fortnight–discharge with instruction to report immediately if any deterioration occurs.

Combination with other Physical Agents:

No form of Electrotherapy should be used as it only confuses the picture.

Exercises: From the beginning the patient should have the responsibility to practise one or two procedures at home–e.g. Arm relaxation, pelvic tilting on a stool, postural contractions. All must be fool-proof! The patient must have the feeling that one takes them into one's confidence and they have a contribution to make towards their recovery.

Articular Manipulation and Traction

Both are frequently used at present and it is therefore important to discuss the relationship with C.T.M. The purpose of Manipulation is to free localised areas from adhesion and make them fully mobile. In many cases they prove a most valuable form of treatment but should never be used without being preceded by C.T.M. Adhesions form by organisation of tissue fluid into collagen fibres. The latter have a tendency to contract. Manipulations are performed in smaller or larger localised areas and therefore may not include the origin of the lesion which has become painless because of immobilisation. The collagen fibres can only be increased in extensibility by increasing the fluid supply. They are a most valuable agent by restoring the cortical pathway for a movement or act as accessory movements to restore full mobility in a joint, provided the extensibility of the connective tissue element of the joint has been restored to its full functional length. C.T.M. should therefore precede articular manipulation which otherwise produces only a temporary relief in many cases. Traction without C.T.M. prior to its application is rather more dangerous, apart from being ineffective in most cases. Manual Traction is preferable to sustained apparatus applied traction. The traction is meant to lengthen connective tissue in muscles and ligamentous structures. As blood vessels and nerves however pass in the same direction, the stretching influence is also applied to the vessel walls and the nerve sheaths. The results are very often disastrous producing thrombosis and other complications. Manipulations, see References (Grieve 1971, 1981, 1983).

The time allowed for the individual treatment session should not be too short—forty-five to fifty minutes should be allowed. This may seem a long period of time but it must be realized that this type of treatment may make all the difference to a patient's life by enabling him to continue working. It should never become a mere palliative.

Most patients report that respiration is easier, and when measured the vital capacity has often been improved. A number of patients have reported that constipation, which has existed for many years, has been relieved and this contributes to the improvement in the general health of the patient. A number of patients feel extraordinarily well and fresh after the termination of the treatment, while others feel comfortably relaxed and tired. In the latter case it is advisable to make arrangements for a rest period after the treatment when patients who respond in this way may go to sleep. This is particularly advisable with patients whose symptoms are due to increased nervous tension. It has been claimed (Teirich Leube, 1960) that the massage has the effect of letting the existing autonomic situation in a patient swing over to the parasympathetic side. Women should not be treated during the menstrual period because the menstrual discharge is increased due to the increase in the pelvic blood supply. Further Contra-Indications are:

Acute inflammatory conditions where a further increased blood supply would be detrimental e.g. acute sepsis, Carcinoma for obvious reasons. A state of Pregnancy would also demand great care and discussion with the Medical Attendant.

The following descriptions of treatments are taken partly from German sources (Dicke, 1953; Teirich Leube, 1960) and partly from the author's own experience. The case histories are all taken from patients treated either by the author personally or by English Colleagues.

When attempting to clarify the use of C.T.M. during many years of clinical experience certain facts evolve. Most lesions are due to Man's inadequate response in his relationship with his environment with the exception of the application of outside trauma such as car accidents, fire etc. They can be divided into certain groups and this arrangement may help during investigation and planning of treatment. The following thoughts might help during the therapeutic approach, particularly when one realises that most of the lesions occurring in Man do not occur in the Animal world. I found the following grouping helpful:

1) Postural Lesions
2) Lesions based on Hormonic or Autonomic Imbalance
3) Circulatory Lesions
4) Lesions based on Head's Zones

The difference becomes particularly obvious in postural lesions which do not occur in the Animal world. An extraordinarily high number of patients suffer from a variety of lesions in the back, sometimes associated with symptoms radiating into the upper limb, even as far as the ear affecting hearing and balance, sometimes into the lower limb. This may manifest itself simply as pain without appreciable loss of function, increasing in severity to impaired and very often almost complete loss of functional ability. Unless we can partially or completely answer the question 'Why' this should be so, we shall not be able to give adequate help to our patients. In most cases we shall only be able to give temporary relief and the patients will reappear at intervals. In a number of cases we shall not be able to give any relief.

The human body is anatomically built in such a way that the trunk is meant to be supported on *4 uprights.* In the process of evolution an upright stance has developed in which the trunk is supported on 2 uprights. Man has to cope with the gravitational situation on the planet Earth and this demands fundamental structural inter-dependence of all elements involved in the upright posture. This makes it essential that the bony elements are grouped round and along a central line of gravity in such a way that a minimum of muscle power is necessary to maintain them in this position. The position has to be maintained often for long periods. It must also be realised that Man is not rooted in the earth like a tree in which the major weight segments are stacked to be aligned vertically. Man is moving continuously and therefore changing the gravitational alignment continuously in thousands of variations at rest - at work and during leisure activities. Upright posture therefore demands the learning of muscular patterns. This learning process takes place after birth and under civilised conditions is very often inadequately fulfilled. Movement patterns therefore become less well developed and the result is an increasing danger of incorrect use of structural elements. Fundamental skills of standing, walking, running, climbing, jumping and throwing are not adequately developed and the body never learns to play with the fundamental force of gravity. We also tend to divide the Human Organism into *Brain—Mind* and *Physical Structure*, forgetting that isolated function or dysfunction does not exist. Misuse may manifest itself in muscle contracture, soft tissue tension etc. but also in inadequate function of the Endocrine and Nervous System. C.T.M. has the advantage that the patient has only to cope during investigation with one sensation, *i.e.* a graded pain sensation. This will provide the skilled Investigator with a much clearer picture of the pathological situation.

After this partly philosophical aspect of Man on the planet Earth let's consider the main facts which are liable to cause an upset in the precarious Gravity Situation. It is essential to consider what is happening to the various structural elements which are incorrectly used, what are the resulting changes in the various tissues, particularly we must find out at which point tissues have become elongated and at which point contracted. Shortened tissue will resist any stretching attempt and this will manifest itself as pain. Tissues such as nerve fibres may not only be stretched but may find themselves in abnormal positions where pressure is inflicted on them. Blood vessels may be compressed and this creates an abnormal circulatory situation which interferes with the optimal function of various tissues. Discs may become unevenly compressed. Unless we attempt to assess the *whole* situation correctly we cannot expect lasting improvement of the pathological situation. Some changes which have occurred are irreversible and we must accept this fact. We can however not afford to specialise in certain physiotherapeutic measures such as C.T.M. - Manipulation - active movements or electrical applications. We must assess the changes which have occurred, be clear on the therapeutic effect of any measure used and apply them in the correct combination.

The first investigation consists of the *Back Inspection*. This will provide us with knowledge about unequal tension in the surface tissues, mobility of tissues and variations in consistency, differences in sensibility, the presence of specific zones, the presence of scar tissue. Further discussion with the patient will provide information about functional disabilities. Further discussion may provide some of the reasons for the discovered changes. The following suggestions have been derived from many years of clinical experience.

1) *Habitual Posture:*

The patient who habitually sits for long periods with one leg crossed over the other. This means that the weight is taken primarily on one buttock, which stimulates the postural reflex on that side, causes increased contraction in all the anti-gravity muscles on that side and shortening of the associated Connective Tissue element. The same applies to the patient who habitually stands at leisure or work with weight on one leg. This will automatically affect the muscles in the lower limb, including the muscles which pass over the knee joint, including the ilio-tibial tract which is one of the most important Connective Tissue structures in the body. Pregnancy, which pulls the lumbar spine into a lordotic position through the weight of the foetus, will cause in many cases shortening in parts of the back and lengthening in the abdominal aspect. Certain occupations demand a stance which causes unequal weight distribution. Stoking demands weight primarily on one leg during a rotatory movement shifting heavy loads. The frequent back trouble in golfers may also be mentioned in this category. Faulty car seats are very often the cause of severe back trouble. Unless the back of the seat is shaped to support the lumbar curve, the psoas takes over as flexor of the lumbar spine and permanently shortens. This eventually severely restricts the mobility of the lumbar spine and the sacro-lumbar junction. This position is often maintained for many hours. It helps, to compare the surface covering of the body to a wet-suit, if stretched on one aspect it forms contracting folds on the opposing aspect. This eventually affects the position and function of organs.

It is quite clear that in many cases the postural position can only be altered to a certain extent. Adequate treatment must however restore the possibility of taking up the correct position and maintain this situation by improving the fluid supply to the connective tissue element in the affected structures and follow this up by strengthening exercises to muscles involved so that the corrected position can be maintained.

Another factor which may interfere with muscle contraction is *scar* tissue. This may apply to the anterior as well as the posterior aspect of the body, *e.g.* carbuncles - old appendix scars, etc. All these lesions healed by forming scar tissue which is fibrous tissue with a tendency to contract, is inelastic and inextensible. It has therefore a different quotient of expansion from true muscle tissue. All these factors combine to prevent harmonious interaction of muscle groups.

2) *Compensatory Lesions*

We must consider that the vertebral column is made up

of 33 bones and represents a very flexible structure. The cervical, thoracic and lumbar vertebrae are connected to one another by fibro-cartilagenous discs and additionally articulated by the joints of the articular processes. The sacral and coccygeal vertebrae become fused and a small movement is only possible between the first sacral and the last lumbar vertebra. At the lower end the sacrum articulates with the pelvis in the sacro-iliac joints, at the upper end of the vertebral column the first cervical vertebra articulates with the occiput. Both these upper and lower connections allow a small amount of movement. There are small movements possible between the individual vertebrae. All these articular structures are made possible by a variety of small and larger muscles and protected by connective tissue elements. The fact that the vertebral column is not a rigid structure but consists of many movable elements explains the occurrence of adaptive compensatory events which take place in case of injury or misuse at any level in the trunk or its connections with the limbs and the head. These adaptive processes can continue until they strike a level where any further adaptation is no longer possible. In my experience a number of frozen shoulders started as lesions in the lower limb or the lumbar region of the back - incorrect postural habits or kidney lesions caused an adaptive shortening of the Latissimus Dorsi Fascia and eventually affected the function of the rotator cuff in the shoulder or vital breathing capacity. Pain on the lateral aspect of the knee joint very often does not represent a lesion in that joint but is caused by an adaptive process which had its origin either in the lumbar region, caused by a shortening of the psoas which prevents full extensor action of the gluteus maximus. Three quarters of the fibres of this muscle help to form the ilio-tibial tract which passes along the outer aspect of the thigh and finally inserts into the lateral surface of the tibial condyle. The tract is one of the major factors in the stability and function of the knee joint. The fascial attachment of the tract may be continued into the peroneus longus fascia and abnormal length in either direction may affect the stirrup action of this muscle in the foot. In women very often insufficient attention has been paid ante or post-natally to maintain a correct pelvic tilt, and its maintenance or re-education. Physiologically the movement in the sacro-iliac joint becomes increased during pregnancy and a slight displacement easily takes place and becomes permanent if not attended to. It must be remembered that the gluteus maximus takes origin along the whole length of the sacro-tuberous ligament and has a direct relationship with the hamstrings, obturator internus, pyriformis, adductor magnus and vastus lateralis. If pain in the thigh or the back is therefore taken as the main guiding factor for diagnosis and treatment, the picture may become very confused. During my clinical experience I have treated three patients where the radiating symptoms primarily affected the cervical region by pain and restricted movement but some symptoms affected the hearing apparatus. All three patients were diagnosed as Meniere's disease. In two cases the hearing was badly affected, all patients showed symptoms of loss of balance - nausea, noises in the ear and gastric upsets. In order to understand these symptoms one must consider the close relationship of three of the cranial nerves, *i.e.* the Auditory Nerve, the Vagus Nerve and the Spinal Accessory Nerve with the muscles and fascial structures in the shoulder region. The main muscles concerned are Trapezius, Sterno-mastoid muscle and Pectoralis Major. Any abnormal tension in these muscles and resulting changes in the circulation in the area will reflect in the function of these nerves and therefore be responsible for the symptoms. The lesion may have started originally by incorrect postural behavior. References: Ebner 1968, 1978; Neuwirth & Gayrat 1959,1960: Travel 1951.

3) *Mental Stress*

This causes an autonomic imbalance, swinging the autonomic tonus over to the sympathetic side, thus influencing the whole circulatory situation. I would like to mention that "Posture" not only relates to physical factors but is also used in the sense of "Attitude". In some languages such as

German only one and the same word exists to indicate both physical and mental attitude (Haltung). The slouching attitude of the mentally depressed is only too well known. The upset in the circulation due to autonomic imbalance may cause a variety of symptoms, *e.g.* various forms of headache, on the other side of the scale the inadequate management of gravitational strains by faulty posture may lead to physical manifestations such as permanent backache because the back extensors are permanently on a stretch. Prior to illustrating the previously made statements by case histories, I should like to stress again that concentration on the areas of pain and functional disability may be misleading and result in inadequate treatment. There are very few lesions which do not involve connective tissue, which spreads like a spider's web throughout the body, and manifest themselves in alterations which can be detected in the back. *Back inspection* should therefore precede planning of treatment. This will be logically followed by using *C.T.M.* to restore a circulatory balance which will permit extension of the connective tissue element in muscle, ligaments and interstitial tissue. This may be followed by *Manipulation* if necessary in order to gain full mobility in individual joints. *Re-education of Correct Movement Patterns* must in all cases precede the termination of treatment. This must be done with simple foolproof exercises, preferably taken from functional every day movements. This permits the patient to include the practice into his daily living pattern and develop correct cortical pathways. Reference: Ebner - Heardman 1982.

PERIARTHRITIS OF THE SHOULDER

The cause of this condition is often not clear; sometimes it is of traumatic origin. The movements of the humero-scapular joint are always limited, and brachial neuralgia is often an additional symptom. It is inadvisable to start too early with the treatment of the shoulder region, especially as relief is often experienced when latissimus dorsi and the subcostal region have been included in the treatment. A painful point is often found at the level of T.2 just below the spine of the scapula. As long as this area proves painful on palpation, the infraspinous fossa should not be included in the treatment. In the presence of severe movement restriction it is advisable to palpate for tension areas over the origin of biceps and the insertion of the bicipital fascia. Both areas may be pain-free but show considerable tension. Another tension area may be present over the deltoid attachment on the acromion process. In chronic cases muscle atrophy may be observed over the posterior fibres of deltoid. In the back, tension areas and areas of swelling can often be observed over the sacrum. During the course of the treatment relief of the lower tension areas often results in the appearance of tension over the trapezius which has not previously existed. See also N.Z. J.O.P.Vol. 3 No. 14 May 1968.

Treatment

The treatment starts with the basic section to which is added the latissimus dorsi. It is progressed by including the scapular borders and pectoralis major. At this point stretching manipulations of the anterior and posterior axillary walls may be added. Should exercises be ordered, these may be included in the form of relaxed swinging movements of the arm to the limit of pain. If the treatment continues satisfactorily, the rest of the back may then be included in the treatment and the strokes in the region of the shoulder joint carefully attempted. By now considerable improvement in the movement range should have been obtained. Any residual restriction will probably be relieved by treating the rest of the arm as far as and including the elbow region.

The patient must practise relaxed swinging arm movements at home.

Summary of treatment

The treatment starts with the basic section and latissimus dorsi progressing to the scapular borders and pectoralis major, infraspinous and supraspinous fossae of the scapula if not painful, and reaction can be obtained, terminating the treatment with stretching of the axillary walls. Later treatments progress to the thoracic section of the back up to C.7, and as soon as possible the cervical section and the shoulder joint are treated. Concentration on treatment of deltoid and biceps is important. Relaxed swinging shoulder movements to the limit of pain carried out by patient at least three times per day.

CASE 1. Female, aged 21. *Occupation:* Coilwinder. On investigation, tenderness of cervical muscles and old tuberculous glands of neck were found. Bladder zone +, head zones + +, right shoulder zone +. Patient suffered from headaches three or four times a week. Right arm elevation was found to be 20 degrees short, external rotation three-quarters, internal rotation one-half, with pain on all movements as far down as the elbow. On palpation there was pain over both shoulder regions, worse on the right than the left, and pain over right lumbar and iliac regions.

Treatment

1. Basic section and latissimus dorsi treated. Skin reaction very marked with wheals over all strokes. All very cutting. Lower back slightly more comfortable after treatment and very warm.
2. Same areas treated. Shoulder ached less, shoulder girdle less tense, less pain on movement, wheals more marked after treatment.
3. Shoulder very much improved, very little pain, headaches less frequent. Same areas treated with addition of scapular and clavicular regions and stretching of the axilla.
4. Pain between scapulae (head zone) still present. Same areas treated with addition of shoulder joint and arm as far as the elbow. Pain over the headache zone easier after treatment but still present on rotation of the head.
5. Pain between scapulae still present. Same areas treated with addition of thoracic and cervical regions. Pain between scapulae improved after treatment.
6. Complained of generalized diffuse pain. Same areas treated. General improvement of pain after treatment.
7. Pain between scapulae persisting. Same areas treated. Pain improved after treatment.
8. Generally much better, no pain on arrival. Same areas treated.

9. Free from pain for almost two days, then pain returned across right trapezius and the medial border of the right scapula. Same areas treated.
10. No treatment for eleven days (Christmas holiday). Pain-free during the whole period until the previous night when slight headache and pain in the right cervical region appeared. Both greatly improved in the morning. Same areas treated, concentrated on cervical and occipital regions.
11. No pain on arrival.

Nine more treatments were given over three weeks to the same areas as before. During this period the patient had three slight headaches which disappeared overnight.

On discharge the patient had received altogether nineteen treatments. Right elevation and internal rotation were full, external rotation three-quarters and slightly painful. Low backache was very much improved, the headaches very infrequent and less severe. General health greatly improved.

ACROPARAESTHESIA

This condition is more common in women than in men. The patient complains of "pins and needles" in the hands, especially when waking in the morning. It is sometimes associated with diffuse pains in other parts of the body. Women during or after the period of the menopause represent a large proportion of the patients suffering from this complaint. The fingers are often swollen in the interphalangeal joints and the patients complain of lack of gripping power. The pain and paraesthesia may be diffuse over the whole hand or follow the distribution of the ulnar or median nerves. Special tension areas are present along the lateral border of latissimus dorsi and over the attachment of this muscle at the inferior angle of the scapula, spreading to the infraspinous fossa. The posterior wall of the axilla is particularly tight. The middle part of the sacrum often appears swollen, while the lateral borders are tense. The area over the posterior fibres of deltoid is drawn in. If the paraesthesia is present on the right side only, the liver zone is often sensitive to palpation. Anteriorly the clavicular area and the anterior part of deltoid are often tense. The treatment should start with the basic section to which is added latissimus dorsi and the scapular areas. As soon as possible the clavicular and shoulder areas are included in the treatment. This will in many cases already give relief of the symptoms in the hand. Should this not occur, it is often advisable to progress to the elbow and if necessary into the hand before attempting to treat the thoracic and cervical sections of the back.

Summary of treatment

Basic section and latissimus dorsi, scapulae and posterior and anterior wall of the axilla. Concentrate on deltoid and if necessary progress into the arm. Special attention to be paid to the subcostal strokes. The treatment should not be terminated before the whole back, including the thoracic and cervical sections, has been treated.

CASE 2. Female, aged 59. *Occupation:* Tailoress. On investigation the patient complained of severe paraesthesia in both hands and legs, which had been present for twelve years. She also suffered from frequent attacks of cramp in the legs. Bladder zone + +, shoulder zones + + +, lymph zones in the legs + +.

Treatment

1. Basic section, ilio-tibial tract treated. All strokes very sharp, hands and feet warm after treatment ("had not been warm for years").
2. Slept well since last treatment and felt generally better. In the morning hands felt "dead." No cramp or "pins and needles" in the legs or feet. Same areas treated.
3. "Pins and needles" in the arms were less severe and less frequent; no disturbance had been experienced in the legs. Both hands and feet had felt warm and the patient had been sleeping well. Same areas treated. All strokes severely cutting and redness marked.
4. Had been generally warm since last treatment. The numbness in the hands began to return after twenty-four hours. The general health was greatly improved and the patient slept well without tablets. Same areas treated with addition of the thoracic section, including the scapulae and the thighs as far as the popliteal space. All strokes were very cutting. the left side more so than the right. During the treatment all sensations of numbness disappeared.
5. The patient had been on holiday for two weeks. During this time she experienced no cramp in the legs; the sensation of "pins and needles" in the arms had been less severe but not less frequent. She experienced less difficulty in holding objects in her hands. Basic, thoracic and cervical

sections treated, including scapulae and shoulders and legs to popliteal space. Some difficulty was experienced at first in obtaining " cutting " sensation in the sacral area. All sensations normal after treatment.

6. " Pins and needles " had been less frequent. Same areas treated with addition of axillary stretching and the arms as far as the elbow.
7. Had felt " very well " since the last treatment, with practically no discomfort. Same areas treated as before.
8. Has had no discomfort in the right arm but experienced occasional slight paraesthesia in the left arm. Same areas treated with addition of the whole left arm and hand.
9. No discomfort for two days, then slight paraesthesia in both hands. Same areas treated as before with addition of the whole right arm and hand.
10. Had experienced no cramp in the legs during the last three weeks but still suffered occasional attacks of paraesthesia in the hands. She still slept well without drugs and her general health was greatly improved.

Eight more treatments were given over four weeks to the same areas as before. During the last ten days before termination of treatment (eighteen treatments) the patient had no attacks of paraesthesia.

PSYCHOGENIC HEADACHES

This is a condition frequently found in patients who live under some type of nervous strain. Sometimes an organic disturbance affecting the body metabolism may have existed in the past; sometimes no organic disturbance can be found. The whole back seems to be tense, and great difficulty exists in moving the superficial on the deeper tissues. The symptoms may be confined to headache permanently present usually in the occipital area, but often extending to the forehead, giving a dull feeling of pain often associated with inability to concentrate. The movements of the neck appear slightly restricted, difficult and slightly painful. Symptoms may extend into the arms with nocturnal paraesthesia in the hands. Particularly tense areas are present over the sacrum and over the paravertebral areas of T.1 to T.7; the region of the ligamentum nuchae is painful on palpation. This pain sensation may be found to extend over trapezius and pectoralis major.

Treatment

The treatment should start in the sacral area and progress as soon as possible into the thoracic region, concentrating on the region between the scapulae, using transverse stroking if the cutting sensation can be obtained. The treatment of this region must be interspersed with anterior strokes over pectoralis major. Further progression passes into the cervical region with treatment of the occipital curved line. The treatment of this region should be interspersed with flat handed release strokes over the forehead. A special attempt must be made to obtain a cutting response over the borders of trapezius. It will hardly ever be necessary to treat the arms. The symptoms usually disappear as soon as a reaction can be obtained over the cervical and trapezius regions. In most cases it will be advisable to teach the patient general relaxation combined with breathing. This should be practised particularly at night when going to bed.

Summary of treatment

Basic and thoracic section including scapulae with emphasis on section T.1 to T.7. Anterior pectoral strokes. Cervical section with emphasis on C.7 and occipital curved line. Anterior facial release strokes. Lateral border of upper part of trapezius. General relaxation.

CASE 3. Female, aged 50. *Occupation :* Housewife (widow). On investigation the patient appeared very tense ; she complained that she could not taste food, felt a lump in her throat, and often felt dizzy. She frequently experienced numbness in her fingers and attacks of headache. She lived alone and felt very depressed. She had a thyroidectomy fifteen years ago, still showed some exophthalmus and saw very badly at night. The back was very tense, the skin hardly movable, the head movements were full but painful. Headache zone + +, maximum pain on palpation over T.1 and T.2 and the occipital curved line.

Treatment

1. Basic and thoracic section treated. All strokes very cutting. Volunteered the information that she felt more relaxed

after the treatment.

2. Several bruises appeared after the last treatment. She felt warm in the back and less " on edge " during the rest of the day. The finger-tips also felt less numb during the rest of the day. Same areas treated.
3. Taste was returning and the lump in the throat less troublesome. The feeling of numbness in the arms had decreased, the pain in the head was less intense and less frequent. Same areas treated with addition of the cervical region, including the occiput.
4. The patient had not felt so well during the previous day, especially as she had been alone all day. Same areas treated.
5. Very depressed on arrival. Same areas treated. The patient felt better after the treatment.
6. The patient was full of complaints on arrival. Same areas treated. After the treatment the head felt much more comfortable.
7. On arrival the patient volunteered the information that her head " banged " less frequently, she no longer felt a lump in her throat, there was further improvement in the sensation of taste and she felt less frequently dizzy. Her whole attitude was much more cheerful. Same areas treated.
8. General impression and treatment as on last occasion.
9. The hands were considerably warmer and the patient experienced less numbness in the fingers.
10. and 11. Condition and treatment as before.
12. On arrival the patient complained of pain in the chest when walking. Same areas treated with addition of anterior chest region.

    The next nine treatments were applied to the same areas. The patient showed a continuous steady improvement in her physical and mental condition.

22. After the treatment the patient was reviewed by the consultant who prescribed three more treatments.

Three more treatments to the same areas were given and the patient was then returned to her own doctor.

After the termination of the course of treatment (twenty-four) the patient's general outlook was very much improved, taste and swallowing were normal, the headaches had disappeared and only very little numbness occasionally appeared in the hands. Her sleeping habits had greatly improved.

CASE 4. Female. *Occupation:* Housewife. The patient was referred to the Physiotherapy Department with a history of headaches with nausea of unknown origin. From the case papers and from the patient the following history was obtained. She lost her daughter six years ago (brain tumour) and two years ago lost both parents within a few weeks. She suffered permanently from headaches with nausea and auditory symptoms such as pressure in the ears, noises such as produced by a tuning fork. Pain was present chiefly at the back of the head, sometimes over the right eye. She frequently experienced a feeling of light-headedness. She complained of numbness over the right side of her face, in the right leg and tingling sensations in hands and toes. She took regularly a nerve tonic prescribed by the doctor and could not sleep without sleeping pills. All investigations by the ear, nose and throat consultant for organic pathology had proved negative.

On investigation the patient complained that she had no appetite and suffered from constipation when travelling. The menstrual period had stopped three years ago but had continued for several months prior to the final cessation. The right lateral area of the calf felt numb. Constipation zone +, venous-lymphatic zone left +, right + +, liver zone +, scapular and occipital headache zones + +, arm zones left + +, right +, menstrual zone showed swelling. The skin over the whole back was only movable with difficulty and appeared very scaly.

Treatment

1. Basic and thoracic section to C.7, latissimus dorsi, trapezius, sternomastoid, ilio-tibial tract treated. After the termination of the treatment the occipital headache and the ear noises were improved, the sensation over the right calf area and the left hand was normal.
2. The relief experienced after the treatment lasted for the rest of the day and the patient slept well with a sleeping pill without waking during the night. On arrival the patient complained of a severe headache, a stiff neck and a feeling of giddiness. Her eyes appeared blurred. Basic and thoracic section to C.7 treated with omission of the intercostal strokes but concentration on the intrascapular area. Trapezius was again included in the treatment which was given in the sitting position. The anterior pelvic region and the anterior subcostal region as well as the frontal area of the face were treated in the lying position. After the termination of the treatment the patient had lost her headache and neck stiffness. The eyes appeared clear.

3. On arrival the patient had only a slight headache. Same areas treated.
4. No headache since the last treatment (two days interval). Same areas treated.
5. On arrival the patient complained of slight tingling in the left hand and slight numbness over the right calf. She reported that on waking she had a slight headache which disappeared on getting up. Basic and thoracic sections to C.7 treated with emphasis on the scapular areas, and the legs as far as the popliteal space. Paraesthesia disappeared after the treatment.
6. No further headaches occurred. Paraesthesia returned after one and a half days. Same areas treated. After the treatment the sensation in the hands was normal, the paraesthesia in the legs had improved.
7. The patient had been away for one month's holiday. She had experienced no headaches during the whole period, but the legs started to become troublesome. The feet were uncomfortably warm and tender to touch. Basic section and ilio-tibial tract treated. During the treatment the skin flaked off very easily. Afterwards the legs felt very much more comfortable.
8. The legs were comfortable during the remainder of the last treatment day, since then the feet felt " sandy." Basic section and thigh treated. The patient was more comfortable after treatment but the right foot still felt " sandy." The treatment was not repeated for nine days as the feet were very uncomfortable and the skin was flaking off. Had during this period an injection of cytamen.
9. On arrival the soles of the feet still felt " sandy." Basic section and the whole of the lower extremity including both feet treated. She felt much more comfortable after the treatment.
10. On arrival the patient reported that she had been very much more comfortable during the interval in spite of a great deal of housework. Same areas treated. The sensation was completely normal after the treatment.
11. Since the last treatment the feet had only occasionally been troublesome. Same areas treated.
12. The patient had been away for one week's holiday. She reported that she had only one very slight headache which soon disappeared. The soles of both feet still felt a little " sandy." Since the beginning of the treatment with C.T.M. the patient's appetite had steadily improved, she

had put on some weight and looked so well that friends commented on it. Basic and thoracic section to C.7, latissimus dorsi and the whole lower extremity treated.

13. The patient reported that the legs were improving and only the right foot felt slightly numb. Basic section and lower extremity treated.

Six further treatments were given to the back and the lower extremity. The patient complained during this period of slight rheumatic pains in the thighs. The treatment was therefore extended to T.7 with emphasis on the liver zone. Exercises and faradic stimulation were given to the intrinsic muscles of the feet.

20. The patient reported that she felt " better than for ten years." The right foot felt completely normal. Same areas treated.

21. The patient reported that she had experienced no paraesthesia in the upper and lower extremities. Back to T.7, including the liver area, and legs as far as the popliteal space treated.

Eight more treatments were given to the same areas.

After the termination of the course of treatment (twenty-nine) the patient was discharged with no discomfort and no headaches.

Patient: Female, Age 52.
Diagnosis: Cervical Spondylitis.
History: July 1983. Headaches for the last 4-5 years, takes 10 painkillers per day.
Back Inspection: Bladder + (Has to get up several times during the night.)
Gallbladder + (Had Cholocystectomy 2 months ago)
Stomach + ? Gastric Ulcer
Posterior Deltoid: ++ (Has always cold hands and feet)
Diagnostic stroke: Very sharp C5-C7
Treatment Progression: For first 3 treatments Basic Section. Perspired profusely. Reduction in severity of headache.

Treatment 4 Progressed to C7 (Headache disappeared during treatment.)

5 Headache recurred 4 hours after last treatment, but less severe. Described head as feeling pleasantly light, first time for 5 years. Progressed carefully to occiput.

6 Sleeping better, perspires less profusely during treatment.

7-10 Periods of relief increasing, reduced painkillers to 5 per day.

Reduced number of treatments per week.

15 Down to 4 painkillers.
17 Down to 2 painkillers.

Patient cancelled treatment during Christmas and New Year period. Telephoned after New Year to inform Department that she no longer required treatment as the improvement had been maintained. Headaches were very infrequent and only very slight. Hands and feet were warm. Instructed to telephone immediately if any health trouble recurred.

MIGRAINE

This is usually described as a paroxysmal nervous disturbance of unknown origin, of which the most constant feature is recurrent attacks of headache, but in the fully developed attack visual and sensory symptoms precede the onset of headache, and vomiting may occur (Walshe, 1958).

The headache usually appears at the time of puberty and the frequency decreases after the menopause. There is often a family history of migraine. The subjects of these attacks are frequently intelligent people found in positions of responsibility, involving hard work and therefore more liable to states of fatigue and anxiety. Physiologically it is probable that vasospasm of cortical arterioles produces the sensory disturbances, especially in the eyes, and the vasodilatation following the spasm produces the headache. Some patients report a feeling of slight general malaise on the day preceding the attack; others feel exceptionally well and bright. Some report a feeling of exceptional thirst prior to the attack. Satisfying this feeling aggravates the attack. The pain is usually experienced in the distribution of the trigeminal nerve, more frequently involving only the upper two branches, but sometimes producing symptoms in all branches. Anxiety and fatigue are definitely factors predisposing to an attack.

Tissue changes are present in all cases in the back between the scapulae which often present a deep drawn-in area. The maximal point is in T.2. See also S.A.J.O.P. Vol. XXI No. 5 Sept. 1965.

Treatment

This starts in the basic section and should be carried out in this area during several treatment sessions. It is very important to give anterior release strokes over the clavicle and the pectoral regions. If possible the initial treatment should be carried out three times a week. As soon as the whole back is included in the treatment this should be concentrated on the intrascapular area. Each treatment must be terminated by subcostal and pelvic strokes. As soon as the tension in the back starts to improve short lifting strokes towards the attachment of frontalis can be added. It is worth while attempting during later sessions the treatment of the face, terminating this with long flat-handed strokes carried out bimanually, starting over the chin towards the temporal region, and gradually finishing with strokes starting over the middle of the forehead and passing towards the ear. In some patients treatment of the face produces symptoms of an attack. In this case return to the scapular region is advisable and no further attempts of facial treatment should be made.

LUMBAGO

The treatment of lumbar back pain of great severity which appears suddenly and makes it almost impossible for the patient to move is discussed under this heading. Disc injury has been excluded by the doctor. It may be due to a focal infection or may occur in patients who are suffering from general fatigue, or it may be of traumatic origin. The condition appears suddenly after an unguarded movement. It may be due to a previous slight injury of the small intrinsic muscles of the back which has passed unnoticed because the surrounding muscles were effective in immobilizing the region and so preventing pain. In other cases deposits may have formed in the muscles due to infection or organic disturbances (Mennell, 1945) and constitute a sensitive focus. The unguarded movement produces the acute pain. The lack of mobility is the result of protective muscle spasm. Improvement of circulation will help to release this spasm and so relieve the pain. Recurrence of the condition will only be prevented if in the case of traumatic injury healing is promoted without shortening of interstitial supporting tissue, and in the case of organic disturbance (*e.g.* appendix or gall-bladder) removal of the cause. Whole big muscle groups appear to be in spasm, in the back the erector spinae group, in the front the abdominal muscles. On palpation localized maximal pain areas can be found in the lumbar region.

Treatment

The treatment should start with the basic section and should be carried out in forward lying, if the normal treatment position of sitting is too uncomfortable for the patient. It is usually possible to make the patient quite comfortable in forward lying with the help of supporting pillows. As soon as possible localized non-weight-bearing exercises should be added to the treatment; the frequently used exercise of standing and bending forward to touch the toes should be banned. In most cases the condition will clear up in a very short time without adding any further regions to the treatment area. Should the condition, however, have existed in a subacute state for some time, with radiation of pain into the thoracic region or down the leg, it may be necessary to continue the treatment by progressing into the painful regions and ensuring that full painless mobility has been re-established before terminating the course of treatment. Teaching of correct postural habits is essential.

Summary of treatment

Basic section in forward lying if sitting is too uncomfortable. Introduction of localized movements as soon as possible. Continue treatment until patient is pain-free by including all areas into which pain may have radiated. This may have to include the anterior aspect of the trunk if the anterior muscles have been included in the protective spasm.

CASE 5.. Male, aged 20. *Occupation:* Agricultural student. The patient was referred to the Physiotherapy Department with a history of having injured his back six weeks earlier while lifting a sack of corn. On investigation the patient complained of severe pain in the right lumbar region which was aggravated when turning the trunk to the left. The erector spinae was found to be in spasm.

Treatment

1. Basic section treated. After treatment the patient felt more mobile and experienced less pain.
2. Basic section treated.
3. On arrival the patient complained that the pain had been aggravated by work (forking). Basic section treated. Relief of pain was experienced after the treatment.
4. On arrival the patient reported less pain during the treatment interval of two days. Basic section treated.
5. On arrival the patient reported that he now only experienced pain when waking up in the morning. This disappeared during the day. Basic section treated and additional pelvic tilting exercises prescribed for home practice.
6. Reported no pain during the treatment interval. Previous treatment repeated.

Two further treatments were given.

At the termination of the course of treatment (eight) the patient had been pain-free for one week during which the entire range of his regular work was carried out. The patient attended three times per week for treatment but otherwise continued with his ordinary work as far as possible.

PROLAPSED INTERVERTEBRAL DISC

Before attempting to discuss any treatment associated with this condition, it is necessary to give a few explanatory remarks. This condition has been exhaustively investigated by specialists such as James Cyriax and it would be futile to consider that the treatment under discussion will produce a spontaneous reduction of a displaced disc. There exist, however, some situations in which the treatment will contribute to the relief or abolishment of pain. According to Cyriax (1950) certain types of disc lesion may reduce spontaneously but leave behind persistent pain. This may be due to bruising originally caused by the disc lesion. Improvement of circulation combined with detailed instruction in correct posture and lifting may permanently relieve the pain. The diagnosis of reduced disc will, of course, be made by the doctor.

Before starting the treatment it is important to ascertain if any sensory disturbance exists. If present, it will indicate the level of the original lesion, and relief of this symptom and relief of pain should soon indicate the effectiveness of the treatment. The areas of sensory impediment and skin tension areas usually coincide.

Treatment

The treatment should start with the basic section and as soon as possible progress into the affected areas. It is important to perform the C.T.M. in the forward lying or lying position, depending on the areas under treatment. It is also important to ascertain that no tension areas exist anteriorly before terminating the course of treatment. In all cases of lumbar disc injury it is important during the posture re-education to stress avoidance of a lumbar lordosis.

Summary of treatment

Basic section in forward lying, followed by treatment of the ilio-tibial tract in lying in all cases where leg symptoms are present. Progression into the areas of sensory disturbance. Re-education of posture and instruction in correct lifting.

CASE 6. Female, aged 23. *Occupation:* Physiotherapist. This patient was referred to the Physiotherapy Department with a history of severe back pain, especially in the thoracic region, which had been brought on by lifting. Prior to the beginning of C.T.M. the patient had been treated for one week with daily traction. This gave very little relief of pain. On investigation the interscapular headache zone was + +. There existed numbness over the area of the infraspinous fossa of the right scapula.

Treatment

1. Basic section, ilio-tibial tract, latissimus dorsi treated. The whole treatment was carried out in the recumbent position and completed with the application of infra-red radiation. The cutting reaction could be obtained with many strokes

only after stimulation of trigger points. The pain had improved at the termination of the treatment.

2. On arrival the patient reported that the previous day's improvement in pain had been maintained and that she had slept better. She had reported back on duty. Basic section with additional thoracic and scapular sections treated.
3. Same areas treated with addition of the cervical section. After the termination of the massage severe wheals over the pelvis and latissimus dorsi could be observed.
4. The patient reported that severe pain only returned after long periods of standing. Same areas treated.

Seven more daily treatments were given, with additional instruction in correct lifting and posture.

At the termination of the course of treatment (eleven) the patient reported that she had experienced no pain after a full day's work during the last three days.

SACRO-ILIAC STRAIN

It is generally agreed that the sacro-iliac joint is a diarthrodial joint and that movement between the ilium and the sacrum takes place in the ordinary movements of the lower limb and the lumbar spine if these movements are carried to the extremes of the normal range. The movements of the sacrum consist of a rotatory movement round an axis which passes through the second sacral segment and the movement takes place in an antero-posterior direction. The joints are directly protected by the sacro-tuberous and sacro-spinous ligaments and the sacro-lumbar ligaments. These ligaments are reinforced by muscles which take origin from them (*e.g.* gluteus maximus), or by large muscle groups which counteract the tendency of the upper sacral segments to fall into the pelvis under the impact of the body weight by maintaining a balanced position of the os innominatum on the femur (*e.g.* the abdominal muscles and the hamstrings). The fifth lumbar vertebra and the iliae are connected by ligaments which blend with the lumbar fascial septa and through these with the muscles of the back. These soft structures will allow a symmetrical movement of the iliae on the sacrum. Should this balanced tension, however, be disturbed by bony fixation of the transverse process of the fifth lumbar vertebra on one side, strain must inevitably fall on the sacro-iliac joints. The restitution of symmetrical stability, if severely disturbed, can obviously only be restored by either surgical interference or by support. In the absence of abnormality of structure sacro-iliac strain can, however, occur under certain conditions. The most frequently met condition occurs in women during pregnancy when the ligaments of the pelvis become physiologically more lax under hormonal influence. To a minor degree this also occurs regularly during the menstrual cycle. During both periods the stability of the sacro-iliac joints will depend solely on muscles maintaining the pelvis in a correct postural position. In both men and women extremes of flexion may occur as a result of heavy lifting; with the knees in a semi-flexed position, the hamstrings are on tension and the load being allowed to flex the back, extremes of tension are inflicted on the posterior ligamentous structures of the sacrum. In women the hamstrings may become adaptively shortened due to the constant wearing of very high heels. The pain associated with ligamentous strain will cause widespread unbalanced muscle tension. Connective tissue massage will help to improve the circulation in the affected areas, which will encourage relaxation of tense muscles and so permit re-education of a balanced posture. Localized and general muscle re-education and re-education of postural sense must be associated with the massage as soon as possible.

Treatment

The treatment should start with the basic section. It is sometimes difficult to obtain a cutting reaction, the stroking finger only eliciting a dull pain, particularly over the more sensitive part of the sacro-iliac joints. Stimulation of the trigger point in the trigonum lumborum may produce a satisfactory effect. Should this manipulation not be successful it must be remembered that the ilio-tibial tract is almost invariably involved, due to the insertion of the greater part of gluteus maximus into this fascial band, the muscle taking its origin partly from the sacro-tuberous ligament. It is therefore often advisable to continue the treatment by the immediate application of short lifting strokes to the posterior border of the tract and progressing to the area round the great trochanter. This will almost invariably produce the desired reaction when returning to the sacro-iliac joint. Should the pain radiate into the whole area of the lateral cutaneous nerve of the thigh it is advisable to continue the treatment as far down as the insertion of the tract.

Summary of treatment

Basic section in sitting if satisfactory reaction can be obtained either with or without stimulation of the trigonum lumborum. If this should prove unsatisfactory, change to lying and treat ilio-tibial tract. Instruction in pelvic tilting in the forward sitting position and re-education of posture (Kohlrausch and Leube, 1933). Instruction in correct lifting, emphasizing the fact that the weight must be pulled close to the body before any lifting is attempted.

CASE 7. Male, aged 40. *Occupation:* Chef. The case papers of this patient revealed that he had been a Japanese prisoner of war for three years, when he had been forced to carry very heavy loads. On investigation he complained of severe sacral pain which had been present during the past two months and which was aggravated by coughing and sneezing. A severe scoliosis could be observed, taking the weight of the body almost completely on to the left leg. No positive Lasègue sign was present on either side. Pain became apparent on palpation over the right iliac crest. This pain was radiating into the right groin.

Treatment

1. Basic section treated. All strokes were very cutting, especially on the left. A marked skin reaction with wheals was obtained. During the treatment the patient perspired profusely.
2. Basic section and both ilio-tibial tracts treated. All strokes very cutting.
3. On arrival the patient reported that he felt more mobile but that the pain had not improved. Same areas treated. The patient reported that all strokes were cutting like " a

dagger."

4. The patient reported that the pain had improved. Same areas treated. All strokes were still very cutting. When leaving the department a considerable improvement in the patient's posture could be observed.
5. The patient reported further improvement in pain and posture. Same areas treated.
6. The patient reported that the pain in the back had improved considerably, but pain was still radiating into the groin when he was walking. Same areas treated.
7. The patient reported an improvement in the pain which was previously radiating into the groin when he was walking. His posture was now fully corrected. Same areas treated.

Three more treatments were given. After each treatment re-education of posture and correct lifting habits were stressed.

At the termination of the course of treatment (ten) the patient was discharged completely pain-free.

LOW BACKACHE

A type of backache is frequently seen in physiotherapy departments which does not seem to be associated with definite trauma such as sacro-iliac strain or disc injury; X-rays prove negative and no pathology of existing or past pelvic conditions can be found. There is, however, usually a history of illness which causes toxic absorption (*e.g.* septic throat) with prolonged rest in bed, or a history of an occupation which is associated with long hours of weight-bearing, particularly standing. The pain is of a persistent but not too severe type, present in the sacral and sometimes lower lumbar region and radiating into the lateral aspect of the thigh, sometimes but not very often as far as the lateral malleolus. The pain is particularly troublesome after periods of rest (*e.g.* in the morning) and is often associated with cramp in the muscles of the thigh after rest. There may be decreased skin sensation in the supply of the lateral cutaneous nerve area of the thigh, but pain sensitivity to palpation over the ilio-tibial band. Special points of sensitivity can be found over the posterior aspect of the great trochanter of the femur, between the trochanter and the attachment of the band on the tibia and fibula, and approximately two inches above the insertion. It might be useful to consider the position of the ilio-tibial band (which is a fibrous structure) in its relation to the surrounding supporting connective tissue. Details of its structure can be found under Technique of Massage (pp. 72, 84). It is not an isolated structure but part of the fascial stocking which surrounds the thigh. It takes origin in a fan-like manner from the posterior part of the iliac crest. Anteriorly it receives the insertion of tensor fascia femoris and posteriorly the insertion of gluteus maximus. Both muscles work synergically when the weight is taken on the leg in walking at the moment when the stepping leg is converted into the weight-bearing leg, distributing the force of contraction of both muscles over the whole thigh and stabilizing the knee joint at the moment of weight transference. In common with other fibrous structures the ilio-tibial band has a tendency to shorten if anything interferes with its blood supply (*e.g.* standing), or if an inflammatory condition exists due to toxins which are liable to set up pathological reactions in fibrous tissue. (Arthritis due to specific toxic origin is another example of such a reaction.) Normally the ilio-tibial band acts as an elastic structure, the elasticity being provided by the two muscles inserted into it. If, however, the fibrous part of the band becomes shortened the necessary functional elasticity is diminished and pain results. As the author herself has suffered from this very troublesome condition, which is fairly common, it might be useful to consider its treatment by C.T.M. and one very simple exercise which has to be practised by the patient conscientiously and regularly. In order to make the stretching of any fibrous tissue possible without tearing it and causing great pain, it is necessary to revascularize it. This can be done, according to the author's own experience, with C.T.M.

Treatment

The massage is carried out in the ordinary way by treating the basic section and the whole area of the ilio-tibial tract.

Additional strokes are added to the basic section by adding short lifting strokes to the posterior surface of the sacrum, passing them from the apex towards the base of the sacrum, and so gradually covering the whole posterior surface. The strokes along the posterior margin of the ilio-tibial band and round the great trochanter are particularly emphasized. They are usually very sharp, but should it be difficult to obtain a circulatory reaction, the trigger point over the trigonum lumborum should be stimulated.

The exercise to be practised is as follows. The patient's starting position is half yard standing, with the hand in extension resting flat against the wall. Feet in close standing, anterior superior iliac spines of both sides on the same level, both shoulders absolutely level. The elbow of the arm in yard position is bent, while both hips slowly lean towards the wall. This causes adduction of the thigh on the wall side and abduction of the other thigh. Pelvis and shoulders must remain absolutely parallel with the floor.

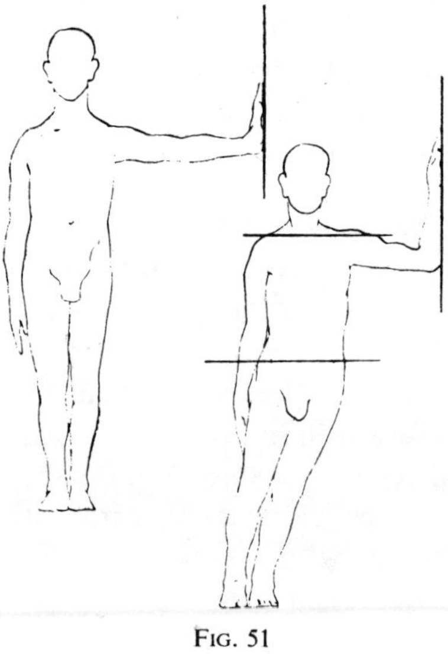

FIG. 51
Stretching of ilio-tibial band.

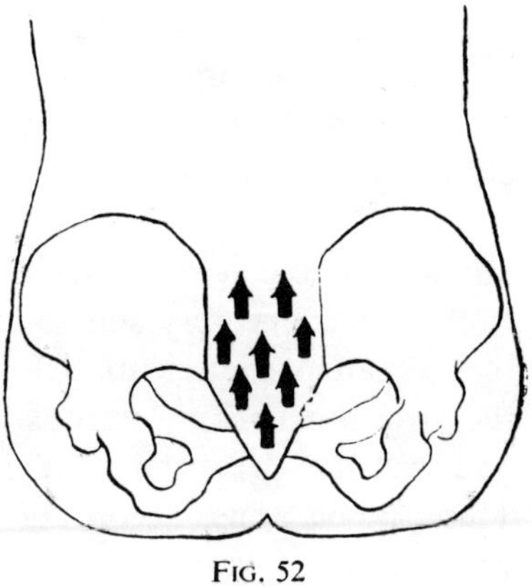

FIG. 52
Sacral strokes.

The exercise should be practised three times a day, repeating it two to three times on each occasion. At first the stretching should only be done gradually as otherwise the pain increases.

OSTEOARTHRITIS

At the present time osteoarthritis is one of the most frequently met conditions in physiotherapy departments. Trueta (1954, 1956) has carried out a great deal of research work which has helped to clarify to some extent the pathology underlying this condition. The first detectable changes take place in the cartilage of the joint. Cartilage is a tissue which does not derive its nourishment by permeating blood vessels. According to Trueta (1954) permeating blood vessels in cartilage are pathological. When a vessel penetrates into cartilage the tissue changes to become either fibrous tissue or, more frequently, bone. In order to obtain its nourishment by imbibition, the cartilage needs intermittent compressions, *i.e.* it must be subject to a pumping action. If, for some reason, this pumping action is absent the cartilage starts to degenerate. In the weight-bearing areas the cartilage will fibrillate and in the non-weight-bearing areas which allow penetration of new blood vessels the cartilage will change into bone and form osteophytes. All the later changes of osteoarthritis are due to this vascular calamity and take place in the form of eburnation and cyst formation. The cause for these vascular changes may be manifold, such as endocrine imbalance (menopausal arthritis), increase in weight (arthritis appearing in middle-aged people), mechanical misuse of a joint (occupational arthritis) and incorrect posture. According to Trueta the pain accompanying osteoarthritis is of a vascular nature. This pain sets in motion a vicious spiral with decreasing joint use, this being followed by disuse atrophy of muscles and increased vulnerability of the joint. This conception of vascular pain might also explain the fact that the referred peripheral pain more often follows a vascular and not a dermatome pattern. The revolutionary concept of Trueta therefore is that the changes of osteoarthritis are not due to ischaemia in the joint structures, but to increased stagnating blood supply.

Treatment

The rationale underlying the application of C.T.M. in cases

of osteoarthritis is that it increases the peripheral blood flow to skin and the other tissues forming the body surface, including eventually the muscles. Exercises to increase muscle strength can therefore be given with benefit. This will increase the muscle protection to the joint and permit re-education of balanced movement. Exercises given with the help of the Guthrie-Smith suspension apparatus and long springs have proved particularly beneficial. The use of long springs allows buoyancy of the suspended part and encourages muscle relaxation which helps to relieve unbalanced muscle tension and also the passive circulatory congestion. The application of C.T.M. often helps to relieve the symptom of constipation present in many over-weight patients. Degenerative changes in joints can be seen by X-ray in most older patients without giving rise to symptoms. The symptoms very often arise as a result of a trivial accident or unaccustomed use of parts of the body. In most of these cases a combination of C.T.M. and exercise treatment can restore full functional use of the affected part.

Before starting a course of treatment it is very important to assess carefully not only the pain and other existing symptoms, but also the existing movement range, the passive range of movement, the pain-free active range of movement and the functional use of the affected part. Investigation of the back may reveal digestive or peripheral circulatory disturbances.

Summary of treatment

The treatment starts in the basic section, progressing up the back as far as necessary in order to reach the segments affected by osteoarthritic changes. Where necessary, treatment should be concentrated on the constipation zone and the liver zone in order to make sure of effective elimination of waste products, particulary in menopausal arthritis. When necessary the doctor will have prescribed a diet for weight reduction and the physiotherapist should ascertain that the patient considers this part of the treatment important. Suitable exercises on the Guthrie-Smith sling apparatus should be added in the department and the patient should be provided with a list of simple home exercises designed to promote relaxation and improvement of circulation in the muscles of the affected joints. Re-education of posture and functionally correct movements is very important. This applies particularly to re-education of walking and standing posture, and advising the patient how to carry out adaptation of household appliances (in women) such as correct height of sink and ironing board. In the case of women it might also be necessary to advise on correct footwear which need not necessarily be flat-heeled, but should avoid very high heels, particularly if these cause incorrect weight impact on the foot. Narrow, cord-like shoulder straps also frequently interfere with the circulation in the upper limb. Should the hands or feet be affected, it will be necessary to progress with the C.T.M. into the limbs. Swimming represents the best leisure activity.

CASE 8. Female, aged 57. *Occupation:* Housewife. Osteo-arthritis of spine with paraesthesia. The patient reported that she had suffered from paraesthesia in both hands during the past twenty-five years. She had a variety of treatments in other parts of the country but had obtained very little relief. She also slept very badly. On investigation it was found that she was suffering from low backache with referred pain into the left leg. There was also pain across the scapulae which radiated into the cervical and occipital regions, and pain over both shoulders radiating into both arms. She complained of " pins and needles " in both hands with frequent attacks of severe cramp. It was found that the general posture, especially in the thoracic region, was very poor. Movements in both arms were almost full, but very laboured and painful. Head zones + +, lymphatic zones + +, shoulder zones + +.

Treatment (*first course*)

1. Basic section treated. Circulatory response could be easily obtained.
2. On arrival the patient reported that she felt relief after the treatment in the lower areas of the back ; the hands also felt more comfortable. She slept well. Basic section treated.
3. The patient reported further improvement in the pain in the back and the paraesthesia in the hands. Basic section treated and the patient taught relaxed swinging shoulder movements for home practice.

4. The patient reported that the occurrence of cramp in the hands and legs was less severe and less frequent; the back felt much more comfortable. Same area treated.
5. The patient had five days' treatment interval and now complained of a great deal of pain between the scapulae. Whole spine up to C.7 treated, including the scapulae. Very tense and cutting over the medial border of the right scapula. The patient was instructed in postural exercises for home practice.
6. The patient reported further improvement of pain in the back and less cramp in the hands.
7, 8 and 9. Same areas treated.
10. The patient reported a great improvement in the pain in the back and paraesthesia in the hands and legs. Head and shoulder movements were easier, the posture was improved and the patient slept better. The pain between the scapulae was still persisting. Same areas treated as before.
11. The persistence of pain over both deltoid areas was noticeable. Same areas treated in addition to the cervical and shoulder regions.
12. Had again a five-days' treatment interval. This produced a sudden attack of pain in the shoulder and cervical regions; the improvement in the lower back and the legs was maintained. Same areas treated as before.
13. There had been no occurrence of cramp in legs or hands. Same areas treated.
14. The patient reported residual pain over sternomastoid, trapezius and the bicipital fascia in the elbow region. Same areas treated with concentration of treatment on the cervical and shoulder regions. The arm region as far as the antecubital fossa was included in the treatment.
15. Same areas treated.
16. There had been a twelve-days' interval due to patient's holiday. The general improvement had been maintained. Same areas treated. The strokes over the bicipital fascia were particularly cutting.
17. There had been a nine-days' interval due to patient's illness (cold). The improvement had been maintained. Same areas treated.
18. Same areas treated.
19. The patient reported that she felt much better, only suffered from occasional headaches, the pain between the scapulae occurred far less frequently, and the right hand still suffered from occasional cramp.

Four more treatments were given. The treatment areas consisted of the whole back up to the occiput, both shoulders and arms as far as the antecubital fossa.

At the termination of the course of treatment (twenty-three) the general health of the patient was very much improved, the back was almost pain-free; the patient mentioned occasional pain over the thoracic region; pain and tingling in the hands had disappeared, only the right ring finger giving occasional discomfort, and the sensations of paraësthesia in the legs had completely disappeared.

Second course of treatment commenced eight months after termination of the previous course. On investigation it was found that a great deal of the previous improvement had been maintained. The patient complained of pain over the paravertebral region between T.6 and C.5; the left side was worse than the right. The left hand showed more frequent appearance of paraesthesia, the right hand only occasionally. Headaches and constipation were still much improved; the patient reported that she no longer suffered from vomiting with the headaches.

1. Basic section treated. Reaction very cutting.
2. Same areas treated in addition to latissimus dorsi.
3. Same areas treated.
4. The whole back was treated to the occiput, both shoulders and deltoid area. Cutting less painful.

5, 6 and 7. Same areas treated.

8. The patient reported that she had not suffered from headaches with nausea since the beginning of the second course of treatment. The paraesthesia in the left hand occurred less frequently. Same areas treated with addition of both arms as far as the antecubital fossa.

9 and 10. Same areas treated.

At the termination of the course of treatment (ten) the patient felt generally much better, the headaches no longer occurred, and the paraesthesia in the hands was only very occasional.

RHEUMATOID ARTHRITIS

Before considering the pathological changes associated with rheumatoid arthritis it is important to realize the fact that very few patients who visit a rheumatism unit will be "cured." It is, however, possible to help the patient considerably and give him the courage and necessary help to live with his disability and continue a useful and enjoyable life. The rheumatoid patient is usually young or of early middle age, of asthenic build, emotionally labile but continuously trying to control the emotions, and therefore finds it very difficult to relax. The patient is predisposed to fatigue and this is probably associated with the inability to release tension. As the highest autonomic control is situated in the cerebral cortex, this cortical tension will invariably affect the circulation in general, but probably also the circulation to some of the endocrine glands (*e.g.* the pituitary gland). This will affect the suprarenal gland which is responsible for electrolyte and water balance, and to a certain extent influences carbohydrate and protein metabolism. This association with the circulation probably explains the reduction in resistance to stress and trauma present in most of these patients. The pathological changes occur primarily in the interfibrillar substance of connective tissue and progress from the inflammation of synovial tissue to perichondrium and articular surface, later producing osteoporosis. The early changes are associated with hyperaemia and increased permeability of membranes, giving the clinical picture of increased joint fluid (swelling). The movement range is reduced, mainly due to pain producing muscle spasm, but can be restored with control of pain. Muscle tone is permanently low due to the disturbed electrolyte balance which interferes with the propagation of nerve impulses. As the inflammatory process progresses to organization, fibrous bands form between the destroyed joint surfaces, which show a tendency to ossify. The speed with which these changes occur cannot be predicted and fortunately the disease is one which shows a natural tendency to periods of remission. This fact makes assessment of physiotherapeutic measures very difficult. The general health of these patients is usually very poor; they often show digestive symptoms and suffer from constipation which is aggravated by the application of some of the more generally used drugs, such as aspirin in various forms. These patients are very susceptible to changes in temperature and usually complain of cold in the limbs, this discomfort often being present to the extent of pain. The question of the medical management of the rheumatoid patient is frequently discussed in the appropriate literature (Hartfall, 1959). This section is only concerned with the problem of applying C.T.M. as a supporting measure which may be of considerable value in giving general and symptomatic relief to the rheumatoid patient. The C.T.M. treatment will always have to be associated with exercise therapy and re-education of functional activities. The effect on the general health of these patients is frequently very gratifying; they sleep better, are able to relax, and the symptom of constipation is greatly relieved. The extensive perspiration very often produced in these patients is another valuable help in the general elimination of waste products. The improvement in peripheral circulation helps to normalize the tension areas usually present in the back and produces a feeling of warmth in the extremities. After the first few treatments bruising often appears, especially in the sacral area. As previously mentioned this should not be painful and does not recur once the superficial tissues have improved in consistency. Should the symptoms in the hands or feet be severe it may be advisable to include these early in the course of treatment. Large infra-red (I.R.) or radiant heat (R.H.) tunnels applied over the back with the use of blankets often prolong the perspiration effect of the massage. These should, however, only be used when it is possible for the patient to rest after the treatment as the increase in metabolic activity results in fatigue.

Treatment

When advisable, the treatment should be carried out in the recumbent position as many of these patients are too tired to sit up for any length of time. As usual the treatment begins with the sacral section. In the beginning the strokes should be very flat and of little depth. The cutting sensation is usually acute and the skin reaction very extensive and deep red. Most of these patients show a distinctive bladder zone and it is advisable to concentrate on the sacral section and the ilio-tibial tract at every treatment session. Progression is made up the back, treating the latissimus dorsi before the rest of the thoracic section. In most patients with severe rheumatoid arthritis it will be necessary to continue the treatment into the extremities, leaving out the joint areas if these should be acutely inflamed. Stretching of the axilla, the palms and the popliteal space often proves helpful. It will often be advisable to treat the back every time but arms and legs on alternate sessions in order to avoid fatiguing the patient; I.R. or R.H. tunnels and exercise therapy should be used, adapting the treatment to the condition of the patient.

CASE 9. Female, aged 47. *Occupation:* Housewife. Previous history: The patient had been suffering from rheumatoid arthritis and gastric ulcers for a number of years. Prednisolone had given great relief but had to be discontinued because of aggravating the gastric ulcer. C.T.M. was prescribed for the period of rest from corticoids. On investigation the patient complained of severe pain and stiffness of both knees and the left ankle. Sometimes additional pain and stiffness were experienced in the head and neck.

Treatment

1. Basic section treated. The patient experienced a pleasant prickling sensation after all strokes. At the end of the treatment a feeling of warmth had spread over the lower back as far as the hip joint and continued to spread over both thighs while the patient was dressing. Stiffness in all joints had eased considerably.
2. The patient reported that the improvement had lasted to the end of the treatment day. The next day the right knee became painful again after standing and ironing for half an hour; the left knee maintained the improvement. Basic section and both lower extremities, including the feet, treated. After termination of the treatment the patient felt pleasantly warm and less stiff.
3. The patient reported that the improvement in circulation had been maintained. She could carry out her work much more easily. The right knee became painful again after twenty-four hours. Same areas treated.
4. The patient reported that she had felt "very well." The warmth in the limbs had been maintained. Both knees were painful especially when walking up and down stairs.

Same areas treated. The pain was considerably improved after the treatment.

5. Same areas treated.
6. The patient had a gold injection during the treatment interval and complained of general diffuse pains. She was unable to hold a cup and could not walk about. The whole back to C.7 and both legs treated.
7. The patient reported that she felt " lovely " until the evening of the treatment day. The upper part of the back and both hands were still comfortable. Both knees and ankles felt painful and stiff. Same areas treated.
8. The patient reported that she had no pain since the last treatment except for brief moments on attempting a change of position or movement. She felt generally much better, had more energy and could move her knees much more easily. Same areas treated.
9. The patient had the second gold injection during the treatment interval. Two hours after the injection both knees became very stiff and painful. This pain had gradually improved but the movements were still very difficult and uncomfortable. Same areas treated. After the treatment the pain in the knee joints had disappeared and good mobility had been restored.
10. Both knees and the left ankle were painful on arrival. Same areas treated. The joints were pain-free after the treatment and the movements easy.
11. The patient reported that full relief lasted several hours; the right knee and the left ankle had since been troublesome. Same areas treated.

12, 13 and 14. The gold injections were not resumed. Same areas treated. A steady improvement in the knee condition could be observed. The ankles were still painful and swollen.

15. The patient reported that she felt generally much better. She had walked on the previous day for half a mile which she had not been able to do for eight months. Both ankles were less swollen. Same areas treated. After treatment almost full-knee extension and flexion to 65 degrees were possible.
16. The improvement had been maintained. A slight stiffness disappeared after a hot bath. The ankle joints were still tender. Same areas treated.
17. The patient had been seen by the consultant. The general health had greatly improved, the patient was eating better

and slept generally well. She enjoyed life much more. The main residual pain was found to be in the right knee and the left ankle. The patient resumed prednisolone.

Six more treatments to the same areas were given.

After the termination of the course of treatment (twenty-three) the patient could follow her normal occupation. The frequency of treatments for the last six attendances had been reduced to twice a week (previously three times a week). The patient was pain-free after each of the last six treatments and this improvement lasted for several days.

LESIONS BASED ON HORMONAL OR AUTONOMIC IMBALANCE

Into this group fall all the Collagen diseases and a number of conditions which are loosely grouped as psychosomatic.

Collagen Diseases

Under this heading are grouped a number of conditions which involve a definite glandular pathology. According to Professor Paul Klemperer from Mount Sinai Hospital, New York, certain diseases are concerned with obscure aetiology. The outstanding common factor is the presence of a systemic alteration of the connective tissue, specifically of its intercellular components. There are however many difficulties present as many questions of "normal" connective tissue are still unanswered. Questions such as the origin of the homogenous ground substance, the chemical constitution of its protein, its relation to fibre formation, the mechanism of hormonal and enzyme control still await clarification (Niebauer 1977). According to Asboe - Hansen (1954), the skin has to be considered as a vital organ which besides other important functions serves as man's front towards the environment. Any alteration in its consistency and therefore functional ability must eventually affect the whole organism. The two most important cells are the fibroblast which is believed to play a part in fibre formation. The Mast cells are present in large numbers, particularly in growing connective tissue. Apparently they secrete important components of the mucinous ground substance, particularly hyaluronic acid. Both types of cells and their activity are influenced by pituitary gland secretions such as A.C.T.H. and supra-renal cortical secretions. Again no clear knowledge is available so far. In most Collagen diseases it has only been possible so far to ascertain the pathological changes which take place but not the causative factors for these changes. The therapeutic efforts therefore have not been very successful. Apart from maintenance therapy such as preserving as far as possible a certain amount of mobility in all structures such as joints and muscles the only drug therapy available at present seems to be large doses of supra-renal corticoids and Potaba. The corticoids produce all the known side effects and are therefore only justified in desperate circumstances. One patient whom I have treated has so far not shown any detrimental side effects from Potaba which proved helpful in swallowing difficulties. The conditions of which I have personal experience are primarily scleroderma and acrosclerosis. I have treated several cases of scleroderma where all the essential tests had been carried out and the diseases have been diagnosed without a doubt. I should like to describe the most outstanding and distressing symptoms. The disease affects the dermal connective tissue and very often the connective tissue in other locations too. In the initial stages the skin is erythematous, red or purple, oedematous or infiltrated and the affected areas are extremely painful. I am at present treating a patient where the disease started in the wrist joints and was diagnosed by the G.P. as tenosynovitis. Gradually however the epidermis grows atrophic, subcutaneous tissue becomes thickened, sclerotic and firmly adherent to the underlying tissues, especially fascia. The skin loses its normal suppleness, elasticity and mobility in relation to the underlying structures. The face is affected in many cases and the tissue changes result in very distressing functional disabilities. The lips become thin and the tissues round the mouth become very inelastic so that the patient cannot open the mouth properly. This produces feeding problems. The tips of the fingers taper and fairly quickly the interphalangeal joints assume a semiflexed position which progresses if not treated by C.T.M. to a flexion deformity. In one case I saw the nails had to be kept below the surface of the fingertips, otherwise the skin of the palm would have become injured. Unfortunately in some of these patients swallowing difficulties appear. (Treatment with Potaba?) One patient whom I saw during a Lecture Tour in 1975 in Calgary suffered from almost unbearable irritation of the skin over the body surface which could not be eased by any form of lotion or even acupuncture. After the first treatment the patient slept for several hours. In patients where the skin over the thoracic area is affected, respiration becomes a problem. After a few C.T.M. treatments, including the Latissimus Dorsi, the respiratory expansion increases considerably.

In the light of present knowledge it is impossible to give a full explanation for these results. There exists however no other treatment to my knowledge which does not produce severe side effects, particularly if the drug dosage is given at a level where for a short time it may produce beneficial effects. I therefore consider the application of C.T.M. given by an efficient operator is fully justified and I hope will lead to further research. Another interesting treatment result emerged from my experience. If for some uncontrollable reason the treatment has to be interrupted for fairly long periods, achieved improvements last for comparatively long periods (up to two months). In addition to C.T.M. the patient must persevere with regular exercises for the affected joints. In the case of hands they are carried out with benefit in warm water, regular breathing exercises must also be included.

Treatment

The treatment starts in the basic section and should progress as soon as possible to include the cervical section. It will always be necessary to treat the extremities if these are affected. During the early treatments these patients perspire profusely and feel tired after the termination of the massage. A short period of rest is therefore indicated. It is essential to review these patients at regular intervals as it may be necessary to repeat a short course of treatment.

CASE 10. Male, aged 36. *Occupation :* Self-employed bricklayer. *Diagnosis :* Acrosclerosis. On investigation it was learned that the patient had experienced increasing pain in both hands during the last ten years. He reported increasing loss of grip in both hands due to progressive flexion contracture in all fingers. He could no longer write. Bladder zone + +, both shoulder zones + + +, full flexion into the palm of all fingers was possible but overall limitation of extension in all fingers was observed. The terminal inter-phalangeal joints were only capable of 10 degrees of movement, the skin of both palms was rough and hard. The face appeared tight and drawn, the hands were permanently cold.

Treatment

1. Basic section treated. All strokes were slightly cutting, the skin reaction marked with wheals. The patient perspired profusely, including the hands. After the treatment the hands felt warmer and the shoulders looser.
2. The patient reported that the hands felt warmer and more mobile for several hours after the last treatment. He had experienced slight cramp in both hands that morning. Basic section and thoracic section up to C.7 treated. All strokes were cutting and wheals appeared. The hands were warm and more mobile after the treatment. The patient perspired less profusely during the treatment.
3. The right hand felt warmer and more mobile for seven hours after the last treatment; the improvement in the left hand lasted for half an hour. Same areas treated with addition of the neck section, the scapulae, clavicles and shoulders. All strokes proved very cutting and resulted in wheals. The patient perspired profusely during the treatment. Both hands were more mobile after the treatment, the right more so than the left.
4. The right hand maintained the improvement, the left hand felt better for two to three hours. The patient reported that the jaw felt less tense; he had experienced occasionally a slight cramp in the left hand but none in the right during the treatment interval. Same areas treated with addition of the arms and hands. All strokes were cutting. During the treatment of the hands, the patient volunteered the information that the fingers felt as if they were stretching out.

5. The patient reported that the wheal marks had lasted for eight hours. He also volunteered the information that he suddenly realized that swallowing was much easier. The left hand now also felt improved. Same areas treated.
6. The head movements could be performed more easily, the palms felt less hard and stiff, the right hand was still better than the left. Same areas treated. The erythema after the strokes was less intense and the axillary stretching less painful.
7. The patient reported further improvement in the neck and jaw movements. Same areas treated. The hands felt warmer and more mobile already on treatment of the basic section.
8. The patient reported that he did a full day's work. The hands felt stiff immediately after work, but recovered fairly quickly. He could handle bricks much more easily than before commencing treatment. Same areas treated.
9. The patient reported that he could now move the fingers individually. He had worked normally for one week. Same areas treated.

10 and 11. Same areas treated.

12. The patient reported that during the last one and a half day's work he had not experienced any stiffness in the fingers. Same areas treated. Latissimus dorsi proved less tense, the fingers were getting thinner.

13 and 14. Same areas treated.

15. The patient reported that he could tackle a job, involving the handling of a steering wheel requiring to be gripped very hard all the time, which he had not been able to do for six months. He experienced no ill effects. Same areas treated.
16. The patient reported some pain in the neck. Same areas treated.
17. The patient reported that the pain in the neck had again disappeared. He particularly appreciated the ease in swallowing and the increased mobility in the hands. Same areas treated.
18. The patient reported that he could now pick up small objects with the fingers, such as pins, which he had not been able to do for at least four years. Same areas treated.
19. Same areas treated.
20. The patient reported that he could now hold a pen and write easily without cramp. Same areas treated.

After the termination of the course of treatment (twenty) the patient's general health had greatly improved; he could lead a normal life and could remain at full work without any ill effects.

The patient was reviewed nine months later and was still at full work and perfectly well.

CASE 11. Male, aged 37. *Occupation:* Clerk. *Diagnosis:* Polymyositis. This patient was admitted to hospital, feeling generally ill and suffering from severe dyspnoea. He could only walk with assistance, complained of pain in the left thoracic region and had great difficulty in elevating both arms, especially the left. During three weeks he received medical and exercise therapy. He was then discharged and continued to attend as an out-patient for a period of a further four weeks. During this period his walking and movements of the right arm were restored to normal. After this period of seven weeks C.T.M. was prescribed. On investigation it was found that elevation of the left arm was still 15 degrees short and the patient was unable to hold the arm in elevation even for very short periods. He became breathless on slight exertion. Previous investigations had excluded heart disease. Venous-lymphatic zones both sides + +, left kidney zone + +. The patient complained that he was permanently suffering from cold feet. The vital capacity (V.C.) with the left arm adducted was 4,000 c.c., with the left arm elevated 2,800 c.c.

Old notes in the patient's hospital file revealed that he had suffered four years ago from a calculus in the left kidney. This had been passed spontaneously some time after the patient had refused operation. Later X-rays proved that the calculus was no longer present.

Treatment

1. Basic section treated. After the treatment the patient experienced a feeling of warmth and well-being. Both arms felt lighter.
2. Whole back treated to C.7. All strokes below the scapula were very cutting.
3. Same areas treated and breathing instructions given. On the left side only upper costal expansion could be observed.
4. Same areas treated. The chest expansion in the left lower costal area showed some improvement.
5. Same areas treated. The strokes on the left side were painfully cutting.
6. The patient reported a feeling of general well-being, felt more energetic and had less difficulty in walking up and down stairs. He also volunteered the information that he was

now able to hold both arms in elevation for a slightly longer period. Same areas treated.

7. The same areas were treated and the strokes to the latissimus dorsi border added. Axillary stretching manipulations were performed with care.
8. V.C. with arms in adduction 4,100 c.c., with arms in elevation 3,200 c.c. Same areas treated.
9. Same areas treated. The erythema following the strokes was less severe.
10. Same areas treated with concentration on the left thoracic section. The shoulders were included in the treatment. After the treatment the V.C. with the arms in adduction 4,100 c.c., with the arms in elevation 3,500 c.c. Profuse perspiration was noted.
11. Same areas treated. Less resistance to the strokes and less cutting was noted during the treatment. This reduction in pain reaction did not apply to the left costal margin, the left scapula and the area over C.7.
12. Same areas treated. V.C. with the arms in adduction 4,300 c.c., with the arms in elevation 3,800 c.c.

13 and 14. Same areas treated.

15. Same areas treated, but both scapulae were excluded from the treatment because a slight skin rash was noticed round the inferior angles.
16. The rash had been improving. Same areas treated. V.C. with the arms in adduction 4,250 c.c., with the arms in elevation 4,150 c.c.

17, 18, and 19. Same areas treated, including again both scapulae. The inferior angles of both scapulae still showed a very strong reaction to the massage strokes. The patient volunteered the information that he slept more deeply during the night and awoke more refreshed in the morning.

20. Same areas treated. V.C. with the arms in adduction 4,600 c.c., with the arms in elevation 4,600 c.c.

Three more treatments were given to the same areas. The reaction to the massage strokes was steadily decreasing in severity.

After termination of the course of treatment (twenty-three) the patient felt very well and was no longer breathless on exertion. V.C. with the arms in adduction 4,666 c.c., with the arms in elevation 4,683 c.c.

CASE 12. Male, aged 35. *Occupation :* Presser. *Diagnosis :* Dermatomyositis. This case history is written in the form of a summary of treatment which has been carried out over long periods, interspersed with periods of rest from treatment with C.T.M. In view of the advanced pathology of the condition the treatment had to be resumed at regular intervals. It was, however, possible to return the man to his regular occupation and full work which was very important in view of the fact that he was comparatively young and the father of several very young children.

He had been treated as an in-patient in various hospitals under several consultants. In spite of treatment with corticoids and physiotherapy his general health had gradually deteriorated and he had lost a considerable amount of weight. Previous physiotherapy had consisted of R.H., faradism to all muscle groups of the upper extremity and exercises. C.T.M. had been started on 17th June 1958.

On investigation it had been found that the skin in the back was almost immovable, the face appeared pinched, and the skin round the mouth was particularly tight. The whole back was painful on palpation, but especially over the areas from T5 to the occiput. Elevation of both arms was possible to 90 degrees but the patient was unable to hold the arms at shoulder level even for short periods. External rotation was found to be one-quarter, internal rotation one-half. The hands showed an overall flexion deformity of 10 degrees; the skin of the palms was very tight and hard. He could handle small tools.

The patient was an in-patient and therefore treated daily. During the first week the treatment was progressed to cover the whole back and the arms as far as the antecubital fossa. The cutting reaction was very sharp and the patient perspired profusely.

1.7.58. Elevation of the arms had increased to 110 degrees, external rotation to one-half, internal rotation had remained stationary at one-half the range. Perspiration and cutting reaction were less profuse. The patient's general outlook had become very much more cheerful, he could maintain a better posture more easily and the skin in the hands was less tight.

31.7.58. The patient was discharged from hospital to attend for treatment as an out-patient three times per week.

29.8.58. The patient felt better in general health than for several years and was anxious to start work. He had gained 11 lb. in weight since he left the hospital. Elevation in both arms had increased, the right arm to 125 degrees, the left arm to 116 degrees, external and internal rotation were possible to three-quarters of the movement range. Reciprocal pulley exercises were added to his home exercise programme.

17.9.58. He developed a skin rash over the back for which the skin specialist provided ointment. The treatment was continued.

27.10.58. The general health was good and he could manage a full day's work quite easily. The rash had disappeared. He could now hold the arms a little longer in elevation. The hands were at present the main trouble. They were painful and went white independent of the weather conditions. The hands were now included in the treatment.

5.1.59. The warmth experienced after termination of the treatment extended over the whole body and lasted for approximately half an hour. The pain in the hands and feet was improving. He stood up very well to full work.

6.2.59. The corticoids had been reduced to one-half during the past month. He had gained a further 1 st. 3 lb. in weight.

29.6.59. He was still suffering from periodical skin rash, otherwise the general improvement in pain, movement range and endurance had been maintained in spite of full work. The treatment was discontinued.

14.10.59. The treatment was resumed. On investigation it was found that the left shoulder zone was + + + +, the right shoulder zone + + +. He complained of pain across the scapular region. The feeling of irritation in the hands was troublesome, the irritation in the feet was greatly improved as compared with the last attendance. The general improvement had been maintained.

9.11.59. The general health was good. The pain in the shoulder region had greatly improved.

18.1.60. On the whole he was very well in spite of full work. His weight was steady. Rest from treatment for three months.

The following summary of the treatment of a patient suffering from widespread scleroderma might prove useful because it gives account of many adverse factors during the treatment period. It also illustrates the fact that it is always worthwhile to attempt the treatment with C.T.M. as no adverse side-effects occur.

Female, aged 49, Occupation: Worker in Sewing Room of a hospital, Housewife

I saw the patient for the first time on 21.3.1975 at her Working Hospital where I assessed her and she had C.T.M. on three consecutive days. She was also shown exercises to practise at home. The treatment interval during the following years was usually one week, because the husband had to drive 40 miles to Leeds on his workfree day. She had however several periods without treatment, lasting up to six weeks because I was abroad and could not arrange treatment nearer her home. On an average she had approximately 35 treatments per annum. She lost very little ground during the treatment-free periods. She went back to work in April 1976 to full duty, including the use of cutting out scissors, and carried out her home work, which meant looking after the house, her husband and his brother.

On June 3rd, 1978 I assessed the patient for a Consultant's lecture as follows:

Face: At first she could open the mouth only half an inch and therefore had great difficulty to take solid food, she also had chewing difficulties. Her general health was therefore not very good. Her lowest weight was 7 stones and 10½ pounds, present weight 8 stones 5 pounds. Patient feels very well. Originally she slept very badly and had almost permanent headaches. Apart from worry, the latter are primarily due to tight occipito-frontalis muscle. She now has periods of several weeks without headaches. She can now open her mouth 1½ inches and food difficulties no longer exist. She can also attend the dentist. She still has a certain amount of oesophageal difficulties.

Right hand: At the beginning the index finger could not be closed into the hand, the rest of the fingers had approximately 40 degrees of functional movement, the wrist could only be extended to the neutral position. At present all the fingers can touch the palm, the wrist extension is approximately twenty degrees. She has a strong functional grip. During the last few weeks the skin in the palm is slightly softer and over the dorsum of the hand slightly more mobile.

Left hand: This is less affected, is fully functional and has a small overall flexion deformity, occasionally she has pain over the wrist, which yields to treatment.

Legs: Functionally only the left leg is affected over the anterior tibial region, consisting of pain and tightness, making plantar flexion difficult. Since treatment began, she has however sufficient plantar flexion to walk normally downstairs and downhill.

Trunk: The skin over the trunk is now hardly affected from a functional point of view. Originally there existed lack of lower chest respiratory function. This is no longer difficult. The patient seems to consider that the weather, particularly cold, influences her condition. She is now however completely reconciled to her condition, she is happy and considers there are many people worse off. I think she no longer presents any psychological problems.

Since January 1976 Potaba was added to the patient's treatment and seemed to have eased to a certain extent the oesophageal difficulties.

November 1979. The above treatment routine continued and the patient lost not a day's work due to her condition.

During the following year due to uncontrollable circumstances the treatment routine could not be maintained, only a few treatments were carried out at a neighbouring clinic. The patient started with pain and functional difficulties in the left arm and right leg. The limbs were cold, she experienced paraesthesia and increasing amounts of pain.

October 1980. I saw the patient again. She had been advised to see a circulatory consultant, who recommended a sympathectomy which was carried out on November 18th, 1980, with a resulting scar above the left clavicle. On December 20th 1980 the old treatment routine was resumed. Although the circulatory surgeon stated that the temperature in the newly affected left hand and right leg was warm to the touch, both limbs felt cold to the patient.

When I assessed the patient, I found that the previously affected limbs were still functioning as before, the newly affected limbs showed the following symptoms: Elevation of the left arm was only possible to shoulder level. Elbow flexion present to 90 degrees only, the whole limb was very painful, the left hand had lost its grip function and the patient complained of severe 'pins and needles'. The patient walked with a limp, the right anterior tibial area was very tight and the first toe in permanent extension. The first treatment concentrated on the very tight Latissimus Dorsi. The left arm was included in the treatment as far as the wrist, heel-toe walking was emphasised and frequent practice of lower costal breathing stressed. After the treatment elevation was only 25 degrees short, elbow flexion almost full and the hand more comfortable. The old treatment routine has now been resumed with approximately 40 treatments per annum. The patient resumed again full work, became gradually cheerful again and has now full functional ability in both upper and lower limbs, the face has lost its pinched look, she has put on approximately one stone in weight, headaches are very infrequent, no swallowing difficulties. The following symptoms may be interesting. Headaches occurred only at the left side. One incident was alarming to the patient: The left Trapezius area and the face became very cold suddenly, patient felt giddy and had to go to bed. During the following treatment these areas were emphasised, no re-occurrence has happened although the left shoulder area is still more sensitive to cold. The parotid gland area in the face and the sub-lingual area are always stressed during treatment of the face, sometimes the anterior area along the sternum is included in the treatment and this has avoided any serious swallowing difficulties. The paraesthesia in the left hand has completely disappeared, the index finger and the thumb were the last areas to yield to treatment with C.T.M. by including the extensor area of the left arm above the elbow into treatment. The patient has been made redundant in April 1983, but leads a happy life, attending to her own household and helping neighbours and friends.

CHAPTER IX

Psychosomatic Lesions

THE common use of this term usually indicates a diagnosis where in the doctor's opinion the somatic lesion is caused by a psychological disturbance.

Having been responsible for the organisation of Physiotherapy Services in a big Hospital Group which included most of the specialised Units, I had some interesting experiences. I hope to share these with the Reader and the result may benefit some patients.

The experience which made me revise my own thoughts was the fact that some patients were referred for physiotherapy by the Orthopaedic Unit—the patient did not benefit from the prescribed physiotherapy and was transferred to the Rheumatism Unit and eventually came back to physiotherapy with a different prescription. After a period of treatment the patient was again seen by the Consultant as the treatment proved not very effective and eventually referred to the Psychiatry Unit. In some cases this patient arrived in the Physiotherapy Department for the third time with a prescription from the Psychiatry Consultant.

I always felt very uncomfortable with experiences of this kind as I consider we are somehow failing to provide help for our patients. This is the reason why I am sharing my thoughts with the Reader who may reject them outright but I hope that the problems may be considered by some in a different light.

As human beings we are not *Psyche* and *Soma* in neatly divided compartments—both continuously interact and react. I am seeing the human organism as a Microcosm which lives and reacts to the Macrocosm, *i.e.* the Human Organism as a whole lives in a certain environment and is equipped to react to the influences and demands of this environment. For better understanding and descriptive purposes we have divided the human organism into a number of systems, sometimes forgetting that all these systems interact with themselves and react with the environment and its demands. The boundary line between the Microcosmus and the Macrocosmus is the skin. This is a very complex structure and at this point I only like to refer to some of its structural elements.

It has a very complex blood supply which helps to maintain our optimal body temperature, it provides the fluid in which other skin organs can function *e.g.* the sweat glands which are vital for the maintenance of body temperature, some pigment cells which protect the body against harmful influences of the sun. The skin is also the seat of afferent and efferent nerve endings such as touch, heat, pain and pressure, some of them belong to the somatic nervous system and some to the autonomic nervous system. All the messages from the Macrocosm are fed back into a centre which is situated in the brain. Here are situated also the highest Autonomic centres which receive and send out in the same way messages to result in functions which are not under voluntary control. In the skull is also situated the highest Endocrine centre in the form of the pituitary gland, communicating through its blood supply with the autonomic centre. This gland with its trophic hormones regulates the function of all the more peripherally situated endocrine glands.

This short summary is not meant to be an accurate description of either the skin or the Nervous and Endocrine Centres. It is only meant as a guide to a certain direction of thoughts.

If the interaction between Microcosmus and Macrocosmus is harmonious and adequate all is well, if however the demands of the Macrocosmus become too great, the Microcosmus cannot adequately respond and the results are all sorts of functional mishaps.

To give a very brief illustration:

A well equipped organism on a cold sunny Winter's day: Skin nerves register cold—reaction via somatic and autonomic nervous systems: contraction via peripheral blood vessels to lessen heat loss, via endocrine system, release of adrenaline to redistribute blood supply—contraction of skin vessels, dilatation of muscular vessels resulting in muscular activity, giving feeling of alertness and well-being. The tension produced is finding an outlet and will make the person happy.

If the demands of the environment are too great, the response will be inadequate. The various centres will still make an attempt but this is inadequate to cope with the situation. The peripheral blood vessels will still contract but the patient will only have a feeling of clammy cold, the muscles will still contract to a certain extent but the patient will only be aware of a certain tension and no productive movement will result—the personal feeling will be one of discomfort.

Many intractable backaches, some sexual difficulties, some headaches and a variety of other conditions fall into this category. Tranquilising drugs, teaching of relaxation via mental pathways, alcohol often prove ineffective as they fall again into the category of symptomatic approach.

Clinical experience in a variety of such cases has shown that it is possible, using C.T.M., to improve the peripheral circulation over the body surface, particularly the costal and sacral regions, which creates a feeling of well-being and relaxation. Concentration over the pelvic region improves the blood supply to the parasympathetic outflow and seems to help to harmonize the autonomic imbalance. In a number of cases this has resulted in an amazing disappearance of a variety of symptoms, a better sleeping pattern and a better ability to cope with the hazards of daily life.

Treatment Outline:

The patient must be treated in the recumbent position in a comfortably warm room. After the treatment with C.T.M. these patients should not be disturbed and rest for at least half an hour. On no account must the stroke produce pain!! Many of these patients go to sleep and should not be disturbed until they wake.

The expiratory phase of breathing exercises should be used to teach relaxation and the patient be advised to practise at home. Simple pendular swinging exercises, experiencing the force of gravity during the swing, prove useful. Other simple exercises may be necessary to deal with individual symptoms. Reference: Ebner (1965) South A.J.o.P.

SUMMARY OF THE EXPERIENCE WITH C.T.M. ON THE PSYCHIATRY UNIT AT BANGOUR VILLAGE HOSPITAL, BROXBURN, Scotland.

Consultant: Dr. A. McKechnie, August 1977

The following summary was the result of demonstrations and talks on C.T.M. given by the Author on the above mentioned Unit. The Consultant and his Registrar attended in 1975 a weekend course given by the Author to qualified Physiotherapists in order to gain personal experience of the Technique and Application of C.T.M.

There was much initial scepticism and this remained for a long time, although it has been somewhat qualified with experience. At that time (1975) treatment regimes in the hospital included drug treatment, physical methods of relaxation and supportive psychotherapy.

Over the past two years approximately 30 people have been assessed and a clinical pattern is beginning to emerge. The presenting symptoms are of physical tension, pain and marked sleep disturbance, both men and women seem equally affected, tension symptoms include: headache, particularly marked shoulder pain, generalised feeling of tension and exaggeration of relatively minor physical complaints with, however, quite definite underlying pathology. Additional symptoms noted have been peripheral vascular impairment, peripheral cyanosis, chest pain often simulating cardiac insufficiency, often excessive perspiration. Drug treatment usually consisted of therapeutic doses of minor tranquillisers, anti-depressants and hypnotics singly or in combination, given at first by the G.P. or the Psychiatrist, sometimes for years, sometimes for several months. Neurotic, reactive or endogenous depression had been carefully excluded. Usually there was a background of a number of emotional difficulties.

Initially only in-patients were treated to control various factors such as drug withdrawal, this proved impracticable and outpatients were included in the trial. People with variable inconsistent symptoms of long duration did poorly, particularly if physical evidence of tension was not present.

Treatment requirements were stringent, such as attendance three or four times a week, which was however arranged flexibly to suit the patient. 15-30 treatments were given. During the treatment opportunity was allowed to talk freely about emotional difficulties with the physiotherapist and also with the referring Psychiatrist, although the latter's contact was minimal. Symptoms were however freely discussed amongst all members of the team, *i.e.* Psychiatrist, Physiotherapist, Clinical Psychologist and Social Worker. As far as possible all drugs with the exception of Diazepam (Valium) were stopped and certainly the total amount greatly reduced. Some patients had been on large doses of anti-depressants for some years and treatment had to be very carefully carried out to avoid exaggeration of side effects. Examination had invariably shown evidence of tissue tension.

Usually after 3-5 treatments the first sign of response was the patient's voluntary information that they slept reasonably well. An important and necessary part of the treatment was the instruction in relaxation. During the treatment it was noted that several quite definite physiological signs were elicited. In some instances there was unilateral sweating, in others disappearance of peripheral cyanosis, feeling of warmth in limbs, disappearance of tension feelings and of persistent headaches etc. There is enough evidence to suggest that inclusion of C.T.M. and relaxation is worth of consideration in the management of severe tension symptoms. This treatment is not a panacea, it only works in certain individuals, it requires skill and an experienced Physiotherapist who has the capacity to listen. It has also proved of interest that in a significant number of patients during the treatment session with C.T.M., some of the apparent emotional blocks to greater personal understanding seem to disappear. This was obvious in one particular female patient: Her symptoms had been apparent since the death of her mother some two or three years before her presentation for treatment. Since then the death of other relatives occurred and she was involved in a car accident. She had severe nightmares of her mother's body as she had seen it after death and had also been unable to visit the family grave. She eventually gained insight into her feelings, and lost her symptoms. It took however a long time and required a combination of C.T.M. as well as supportive psychotherapy.

Due to a small grant and the devotion of the staff at the Unit it was possible to carry out a Pilot Study about the treatment of "Anxiety States" by C.T.M. and psychotherapy. This study was carried out under research conditions. Reference: McKechnie 1983.

Personal Experience of the Author: I have treated a number of patients with C.T.M., respiratory exercises and instruction in relaxation. All these patients suffered from severe back trouble, especially in the cervical and shoulder region and very frequent attacks of headache. The headaches usually disappeared if the C.T.M. strokes were emphasised over the lower part of the occiput, the upper part of trapeius and the upper part of the face, particularly the frontalis area. It must be remembered that the name of the muscle which covers the head is called Occipito-Frontalis. It attaches along the curved line of the occiput—over the whole skull to the frontal bone. Reference: Ebner (1978), Reference: Neuwirth and Gayal (1959,1960).

Patient: Female, Age 32

History and Diagnosis: Has had headaches daily for the last one and a half years, complains of pins and needles in left arm and leg. Has been fully investigated for headaches. No obstetric abnormalities. Gives account of broken marriage. Has a history of Depression. Sleeps very badly. Treatment requested by Consultant C.T.M.

Back Inspection: Arterial area + (suffers from cold feet). Interscapular area ++ (headaches for 1½ years daily)

Progression of Treatment:

First two treatments Basic section, third treatment progressed to T 12.

Treatment 4 very carefully progressed into interscapular area.
5 reported improved sleeping pattern, same areas treated.
6 two days without headaches. Same areas treated.
7-10 Gradually worked up to occipital curved line. (very tight)
11 Headaches only occasionally and very slight. Pins and needles in arm and leg practically disappeared.
12-14 Sleeps well, feels very well and is cheerful, no arm or leg complaint. Treatment: Whole back to occipital line incl.

Two further treatments given, discharged with instruction to contact the Physiotherapy Department immediately if any disability occurs. January 1984 no contact made by Patient or G.P. (3 months).

CHAPTER X

Peripheral Vascular Disease

THIS group contains a great variety of conditions resulting in disturbance of the circulation in the limbs. This disturbance may occur in the venous part of the circulation (*e.g.* varicose veins) or in the arterial part of the circulation. Although venous circulatory disturbances may benefit very much by the application of C.T.M., especially if they are accompanied by ulceration, the conditions discussed under this heading will be primarily disturbances in the arterial part of the circulation. The results obtained with the modern methods of application originated by Bisgaard in venous disturbances are very satisfactory and there does not seem to be any need to venture into new fields of treatment in most cases. The usually applied treatment methods in arterial disturbances, however, seem to be less satisfactory and very often do not even provide symptomatic relief for short periods. The functional insufficiency may be due to degenerative changes in the arterial vascular system (*e.g.*, arteriosclerosis, endarteritis obliterans), or to functional disturbances of the vascular control (intermittent claudication, Raynaud's disease, acrocyanosis). Improvement can, of course, only be expected in so far as changes which have occurred are still reversible or the obliterated vessels can be replaced by the establishment of a collateral circulation. Vasodilatation can occur due to nervous influences and in response to blood-borne chemical stimuli (Hill and Wilson, 1950). Both can be influenced by C.T.M. For these conditions C.T.M. will therefore often be the preferential treatment, especially as German investigators (Völker and Rostovsky, 1949) have proved that the results obtained are at least as good as, and in many cases better than, the application of vasodilator drugs.

Since the last revision of this book the Author has realised that the group "Circulatory Lesions" comprises a much greater number of conditions of widely different aetiology and pathogenesis as previously anticipated. It is not only the distribution which is affected but also the composition of the fluid which bathes the tissue cell. One of the most frequent complications is diabetes. This is also one of the most dangerous complications as it very often leads to gangrene of the extremity (leg) and amputation of the limb. It is only a question of time until the second limb is affected with the disease, followed by amputation. It may be a coincidence and certainly demands further investigation but in three cases known to the Author, the insulin deficiency improved remarkably. As usually not all the insulin producing cells are affected, the better blood supply provided by C.T.M. to the pancreas zone, may produce better function of the remaining cells. The case described at the end of this chapter was a Diabetic. Severe anaemia also showed in some patients, apart from circulatory disturbances, osteoporosis of the upper femoral region with disturbances in the function of the hip joint. This may explain the comparatively high failure rate of hip-replacement operations which are carried out under otherwise excellent conditions.

On investigation the connective tissue changes in the back and in the proximal part of the affected limbs are very obvious. The severity of the changes is a reliable guide to the severity of the condition. The skin of the affected limbs shows changes in colour; it may be greyish-white or bluish-red, depending on the predominance of vasospasm or stasis. The patient often complains that the skin over the sacrum and the buttocks or over the shoulder region feels too tight and restrictive to movement. The cutaneous and subcutaneous tissues are closely adherent and the moving finger encounters strong resistance. It is therefore essential to commence work with very short strokes.

The patient's sensation and skin reaction are different from the reactions experienced in other conditions. It is very difficult in the initial stages to obtain a scratching or cutting reaction; the patient often only reports the sensation of slight pressure under the stroke which is, however, not painful. The reddening of the skin is at first very faint and only appears after several strokes have been applied over the same area. As the treatment sessions progress, the skin reaction takes a shorter time to appear and gradually changes in colour, *i.e.* it becomes red and dark-red until finally a wheal results. Gradually also the sensation changes from a slight pressure sensation to scratching and eventually to severe cutting. From this point onwards the reaction in further treatments follows the previously discussed pattern, *i.e.* simultaneously with the decrease in the severity of the cutting sensation, the skin reaction becomes less violent and eventually follows the pattern of reaction of normal skin. The course of treatment can be terminated when the stroke reaction is slightly cutting, the skin reaction slightly red and diffuse and when it has disappeared after a short period.

The decrease of the tissue tension in the back coincides with a decrease of pain and spasm in the limbs and improvement of functional endurance. The colour of the skin also approaches the colouring of the rest of the body.

INTERMITTENT CLAUDICATION

This is a symptomatic condition which occurs in two main groups of patients:

1) Patients who are usually advanced in years and often show general signs of arteriosclerosis. The patient has no discomfort except on walking and complains that the extremities, more often the legs, sometimes both hands and legs, feel cold. After walking a variable distance, depending on the severity of the condition, pain and fatigue are felt. The patient experiences a cramplike feeling, and rest becomes imperative. After a short rest the patient can continue but the distances covered become increasingly shorter. The patients are otherwise often in good health and the forced inactivity is therefore very distressing. Although the affected limb feels cold to the patient and is often pulseless, the skin temperature when measured, may not be dif-

ferent from the unaffected limbs. (Bach 1950) In some of these patients the vessels affected primarily are much higher up such as the branches of the abdominal aorta.

Experimental investigation seems to confirm the fact that not only the arteries but also the capillaries are affected and vaso-dilatation produced by any method must produce an increase in the peripheral vascular bed. (Hill and Wilson 1950). Vascular surgery is therefore very often not very effective, and it is on this basis that the favourable results experienced by the Author using C.T.M. may be explained.

2) Patients who usually belong to a younger age group, the outstanding symptom again is intermittent claudication but the general health of the patient is less good. They usually complain of other functional disturbances, primarily gastric and digestive symptoms. In my experience these patients usually cannot relax and often are heavy smokers. The Back Inspection shows frequently gastric or other digestive zones, apart from the circulatory zones. The vascular changes therefore may be due to disturbances of the vascular nervous control. I consider the smoking habit is a result of the existing tension state. Unfortunately nicotine aggravates the circulatory condition as it affects the synapses of the autonomic fibres, the parasympathetic synapses are however more affected than the sympathetic ones. The vaso-constrictor influence of the sympathetic nervous system on the capillary bed therefore increasingly prevails. These patients must therefore be helped to give up smoking or drastically reduce it.

Treatment

C.T.M. in forward lying. The basic section, if necessary up to T.7, only short strokes should be used at first and repetition up to ten times may be necessary. In spite of using Trigger points, it may be impossible at first to obtain a scratching reaction or an erythema. In spite of the lack of sensory or visible reaction the patient often experiences a feeling of warmth in the affected limb. It is inadvisable to progress too quickly into the foot as circulatory channels may not yet have opened. Painful areas such as the calf should be avoided until a reaction can be obtained. The sensitivitiy of the calf area may be explained by the fact that the intra-muscular anastomosis of blood vessels varies considerably in different muscles. Both soleus and gastrocnemeus seem to have a very vulnerable blood supply (Blomfield 1950) and this may explain why the disability becomes particularly evident in this muscle group. During a progressive course of treatment this tenderness disappears and treatment of this area can be resumed. Too early C.T.M. treatment of areas with faulty or painful reaction may make the patient very uncomfortable during the following night and does *not* produce any beneficial results. The hamstring area should be treated prior to the calf. If the upper limbs are affected the C.T.M. treatment must be progressed as far as C1 and in the presence of tension headaches, the occiput and upper face areas also included. The degree of recovery of all tension areas is a very good guide to the correct application of C.T.M.

All these patients must have at least half an hour's rest after treatment. Prior to the beginning of the C.T.M. treatment it will be advisable to teach lower costal and abdominal breathing in the lying position with head and shoulders supported on one or two soft pillows to obtain relaxation of the abdominal muscles. (Warning the patient not to practise these exercises more than three or four times consecutively in order to avoid oversaturation with oxygen.) During the day practise in sitting. Simple circulatory exercises will prove helpful to the patient, *e.g.* elbow flexion and extension, hip and knee flexion, ankle rolling etc.

The second group of patients, complaining of intermittent claudication and consisting usually of a much younger age group, demands particularly careful investigation in order to find additional functional disabilities, as previously described. Apart from specific zones relating to organs, it will be found that large fascial structures such as the latissimus dorsi fascia, the ilio-tibial tract, the trapeius fascia, are very tense. The C.T.M. treatment as described above must therefore pay careful attention to these structures. The additional treatment of the anterior subcostal and costal areas proves often very rewarding. When treating the upper trapezius area an amazing release of tension is often achieved by changing the treatment position to sitting and interspersing the posterior strokes with anterior release strokes. For these the whole flat hand of the operator is used, starting at the lower border of pectoralis major and carrying the flat-handed stroke up over the clavicular and shoulder area (pathway of vagus nerve) and ending over the posterior aspect of deltoid. For the treatment of the lower extremity the lying and forward lying positions are again resumed. Breathing exercises, circulatory exercises and relaxation should only be checked during the treatment period but otherwise be carried out by the patient at home.

The establishment of a more effective collateral circulation must include the whole body surface. It is also essential to increase muscle endurance. The most effective general exercises are swimming and walking. These patients should be encouraged to take walks of increasing length, particularly on turf. These patients must also rest at least half an hour after treatment. It is essential in the treatment of this condition to keep records of the distance which can be covered or the amount of work which can be done without discomfort.

Summary of the treatment of a patient Group 2.

Female, aged 48, Housewife. This patient had for several years suffered from indigestion which eventually was diagnosed as a stomach ulcer and treated surgically. No further gastric trouble was experienced. The patient played golf as her recreational activity. She played again regularly after the recovery from the gastric ulcer, at first greatly enjoying the activity. Gradually she discovered it became increasingly difficult to play a full round. Eventually the play of two holes produced severe symptoms of claudication.

On investigation the following zones were noted: Arterial zones in both legs ++, right arm ++, left arm +. Stomach zone ++. The patient was previously known to the Author. During the first treatment the following information was gained: The patient was greatly worried about the health of her husband, she was also greatly worried about her daughter's marriage, who no longer lived with her husband and had the care of two small children. She smoked about 40 cigarettes per day. She had at first three treatments per week, reduced gradually to one treatment per week, altogether twenty C.T.M. treatments were given. Relaxation and breathing exercises were included. The patient had the willpower to stop smoking at once, satisfying the urge to smoke at first with peppermints. She continued to play golf over increasing distances, a full round was possible after two months. She learned to manage the difficulties in her life which eventually included the death of her husband. She is still playing regular golf.

CASE 13. Female, aged 36. *Occupation :* Housewife. This patient's case history revealed that she had been treated six years ago for disc lesion (?) with a plaster of Paris jacket. The following year a carpal tunnel decompression operation had been performed in the left hand. She complained of a burning sensation in the upper arms and " pins and needles " in the hands. These sensations of paraesthesia had been present for six months. She could not walk for more than one mile, when the ankles became painful and felt as if they were " locking." She had to rest before she could resume walking.

On investigation the following zones were noted: Bladder zone + +, left shoulder zone + +, right shoulder zone +. The treatment was carried out twice weekly.

Treatment

1. Basic section treated. The back was very tense and all strokes were very cutting. Marked skin reaction with wheals. After the treatment the patient felt warm and braced up.
2. The patient reported that she felt " on top of the world " for one hour after the last treatment with no discomfort or pain. The pain returned later in the lower back and buttocks. She had a completely undisturbed night. Basic section treated, with marked wheal reaction.
3. The patient reported that she had no discomfort for four days; two nights were slightly disturbed by the sensation of " pins and needles " in the hands. She had, however, felt slightly bilious during the last three days. The whole back treated to C.7. All reactions very cutting but less wheal appearance. Profuse perspiration occurred during the treatment.
4. The patient reported that she felt " grand " since the last treatment. Only one night had been disturbed by the appearance of a slight " pins and needles " sensation.

The whole back and neck, scapulae and shoulder joint area treated. Marked wheals appeared in the shoulder region.

5. The patient reported three short periods of "pins and needles" during the last night. Same areas treated.
6. The patient reported that she had a short attack of not very severe pain in the lower back and down both arms on the previous day. Same areas treated, with addition of both axillae and both arms as far as the deltoid insertion.
7. Same areas treated, with addition of the whole of the upper arm and the antecubital fossa.
8. The patient had no sensory disturbances since the last treatment. Same areas treated with addition of the forearms.
9. Same areas treated.
10. The patient reported that she had experienced no severe pain or discomfort during the past two weeks. The treatment was modified to skin rolling only (menstrual period).
11. Same areas treated (skin rolling only).
12. The patient reported that she had experienced no pathological symptoms of any kind. Treatment to all areas resumed.

Two more treatments to the same areas were given.

After termination of the course of treatment (fourteen) the patient had been completely symptom-free for three weeks.

CASE 14. Female, aged 57. *Occupation:* Housewife; has helped husband in butcher's shop. The patient's case papers revealed that six years ago in hospital she had been treated with iron for severe anaemia. Since then she had developed rheumatoid arthritis, intermittent claudication and extensive psoriasis.

Prior to the present course of treatment with C.T.M. she had been in hospital for five weeks. ACTH drip produced considerable improvement of the arthritic condition. Both wrists still showed a condition of mixed arthritis which was treated with ultra-short-wave and wax to the hands. After this treatment the hands gave little discomfort and showed good functional ability. The most distressing symptom for the patient was the inability to walk for more than 20 to 30 yds. without having to rest. Daily sinusoidal baths had produced no improvement in the condition.

On investigation for C.T.M.: Bladder zone +, arterial zones in both legs + (slightly more on the left), liver zone +.

Treatment

1. Basic section and both thighs as far as the popliteal space treated. A slight reddening reaction and wheal formation

was obtained. Two and a half hours after this first treatment the patient could still walk 60 yds. without rest period.

2. On the following day the patient could still walk the same distance without discomfort. Same areas treated. Two and a half hours after termination of treatment the patient could walk 80 yds. without feeling tired.
3. Same areas treated. The patient was discharged from hospital, taking prednisolone regularly.
4. Three weeks later the C.T.M. treatment was resumed in the patient's home. The improvement in walking distance had been maintained. The patient suffered from severe cramp during the night and could only get a few hours sleep with the help of sleeping tablets. She suffered from frequent attacks of occipital headaches and flushes in the face. Both feet were cold and blue, the dorsalis pedis artery was not palpable. Pain was present on palpation over both calves. Basic and thoracic section, latissimus dorsi, and legs as far as the knee treated, with stretching of the popliteal space. After the treatment the feet were warm and the veins on the dorsum filled. At this stage it was planned to carry out the treatment twice a week at home.
5. The patient reported that she could now walk for twenty minutes at a slow pace without rest. The nights were still disturbed by cramp in the legs and flushes in the face. On arrival the feet were warm. The whole back to C.7, latissimus dorsi, and the whole lower extremity including the feet treated, with stretching of the popliteal space and the soles of the feet.
6. The patient had been away for the week-end and could walk for thirty minutes without rest. The nights were less disturbed, and the flushes less frequent but not less severe. She reported bruises after the last treatment over the sacrum and the latissimus dorsi border. The feet had been warm since the last treatment. Same areas treated with addition of strokes along the anterior border of trapezius. The leg strokes were very cutting but with only faint reddening.
7. The patient reported that she felt well and had started to work short periods in the shop. Same areas treated with addition of the shoulders and the arms as far as the antecubital fossa.
8. The patient reported that she experienced no ill effects from working short periods in the shop. The calves no longer

felt fatigued, and the feet only now started to feel tired. Sleep was improving. Same areas treated with addition of the soles of the feet and the toes. Toe strokes extremely sharp.

9. There had been a three-weeks' treatment pause. During this interval the walking distance had been maintained, the patient no longer suffered from cramp in the calves and flushes had become more frequent during the last week. Wrists were slightly troublesome but responded to Kaolin treatment. The whole back, arms and hands, legs and feet treated.

10. The patient reported further improvement in walking distance. She managed to go for an afternoon's shopping, walking slowly with only a longer interval for tea. Same areas treated.

The treatment frequency was now reduced to once a week. Seven further treatments were given to the same areas.

18. The patient reported that she was now able to do all necessary work in the house and shop without having to rest. She could join in family excursions without any discomfort. The walking time was thirty to forty minutes without fatigue when walking not too quickly. The feet were always warm, independent of climatic conditions. She had undisturbed nights and felt very well. Flushes were less frequent and less severe. The wrists were sometimes troublesome. Prednisolone was reduced by the consultant with planned further reduction and eventual discontinuation.

Twelve further treatments to the same areas were given.

31. The patient felt no ill effects from the reduction of prednisolone which had now been discontinued. She could walk for an hour at reasonable speed without rest. The feet were always warm in spite of wintry conditions.

The treatment had now been reduced to intervals of approximately two weeks. Longer intervals up to four weeks due to holidays had produced no deterioration of the condition.

P.S. During the past 12 years the author and several colleagues have treated a number of cases with sometimes amazing results. One case in particular is worth mentioning. A female patient, suffering from inoperable stoppage of the abdominal aorta (arteriogram) with resulting gangrene of the foot. The patient had not walked for the past 2 years. She was eventually discharged with the foot healed, afterwards 2½ toes were enucleated because all tissues were completely dead. The patient could walk unassisted and went unassisted to Canada where she spent the winter. She is being regularly reviewed and receives a booster dose of approximately 4 weeks duration once a year.

Recent Case History: Female 82 years old.

History and Diagnosis.

Peripheral Vascular Disease with bilateral claudication. No pulse below left femoral artery, which is occluded, no pulses over the rest of both legs. Walking Distance 75 yards, no stairs or uphill walking possible because of immediate pain. Stopped smoking 27 years ago, had coronary (prophylactic) by-pass operation in U.S.A. because of slight chest pain.

Back Inspection:

Bladder + + (gets up twice per night,) Gallbladder +, Stomach + (dislikes fatty food and suffers from Heartburn), Arms + + Fingers go white in winter, Lumbar Back + (suffers from continuous Backache).

Progress of Treatment:

First 4 treatments: Basic Section, gradually progressing into lower legs. Walking felt easier, but left Hallux was still painful and red.
After 6 treatments: All toes are better colour, no shooting pains during the night in bed, can manage stairs now easily.
After 8 treatments: No backache, feels well and sleeps well.
After 12 treatments: Left Hallux looks and feels normal.
After 24 treatments: Discharged. Can do all her shopping and housework.
Walking Distance: 300 yards.
Toe Temperature: Pre-Treatment L. Hallux: 26.6° R. Hallux: 28.8°
Post Treatment L.H. 33.6° R.H. 28.8°

RAYNAUD'S PHENOMENON

This condition may be defined as intermittent pallor or cyanosis of the extremities of varying intensity. This symptomatic interference with the peripheral circulation is precipitated by cold and does not usually show blockage of the large arteries. It may occur in various forms, for example, in normal persons on exposure to cold, in association with hereditary cold extremities, sometimes in workers with vibrating tools, and sometimes as the precursor of other circulatory disorders, such as sclerodactyly or thromboangiitis obliterans. The specific diagnostic sign is the intermittency of the symptoms (Hill and Wilson, 1950). It is usually assumed that the interference with the peripheral circulation is due to reflex spasm. In severe cases the interference with the peripheral circulation may lead to tissue breakdown, particularly during the cold season.

The peripheral skin usually shows a greyish-blue tint and the whole back shows increased tension in the affected segments, particularly noticeable in the cervical and upper thoracic segments if the hands are primarily affected, and in the lower lumbar and sacral segments if the lower limbs are affected.

Treatment

As in other pathological conditions due to arterial spasm, the reactions following the application of the massage strokes are different. It is far more difficult to obtain a cutting reaction and this can often only be achieved after a number of applications. Strokes over special trigger points, such as the border of latissimus dorsi, trigonum lumborum, axilla, the posterior border of the ilio-tibial tract and the great trochanter, the adductor hiatus, the inferior angle of the scapula, and the anterior border of trapezius, are often necessary to obtain a slight reaction initially. The increase in the intensity of the cutting reaction usually coincides with an increase in the intensity of the skin reaction. Later on the reaction follows the normal course of progress, *i.e.* it becomes less severe as the circulatory condition improves. This represents a very good guide to the success of the treatment.

German authors (Teirich-Leube, 1960) claim that a change of autonomic reaction towards the parasympathetic side takes place and for these patients some rest after treatment is recommended. Symptomatic improvement of circulation is often noticeable after a small number of treatments, but it is advisable to continue the treatment for several weeks after this has taken place.

It may be necessary to repeat a course of treatment once a year before the beginning of the winter season. Success of treatment depends on the amount of permanent damage which may have occurred in the vessel walls. In many cases C.T.M. alone will result in great improvement of the condition. Should the doctor in charge of the case prescribe drugs, the application of C.T.M. will enhance the effect of these.

Summary of treatment

The treatment should be started in the back in the sitting position whenever this is possible. Long strokes are inadvisable as the back shows much increased tension. Short, slow strokes which will demand a certain amount of pressure must first increase the mobility of the tissues in the back. Six to ten treatments may be necessary before this is achieved. The treatment should at first be concentrated on the lumbar, sacral and buttock regions. Patients often report irritating sensations in the more peripheral distribution of the segments under treatment (*e.g.*, calf or foot). This will make it advisable to reduce the speed of the stroke as far as possible. Freedom from this irritation will be the result. Patients very often report an increase in the feeling of warmth in the extremities when tension in the back has been decreased. At this point it may be advisable to progress the treatment into the extremities, especially if ulceration has previously occurred in peripheral areas.

CASE 15. Female, aged 32. *Occupation*: Weaver. The patient complained that as far as she could remember her fingers had frequently "gone dead." She often dropped objects held in her hands. On investigation: Venous-lymphatic zone +, scapular headache zone +, arm zones + +.

Treatment

1. Basic section, latissimus dorsi border treated. It was difficult to obtain a circulatory reaction and the trigger point over the trigonum lumborum had to be stimulated.

2 and 3. Same areas treated.

4. The patient reported that the circulation in the hands had improved. Same areas treated.
5. Same areas treated.
6. The patient reported that the hands felt less frequently "dead" and that she now was able to hold objects without dropping

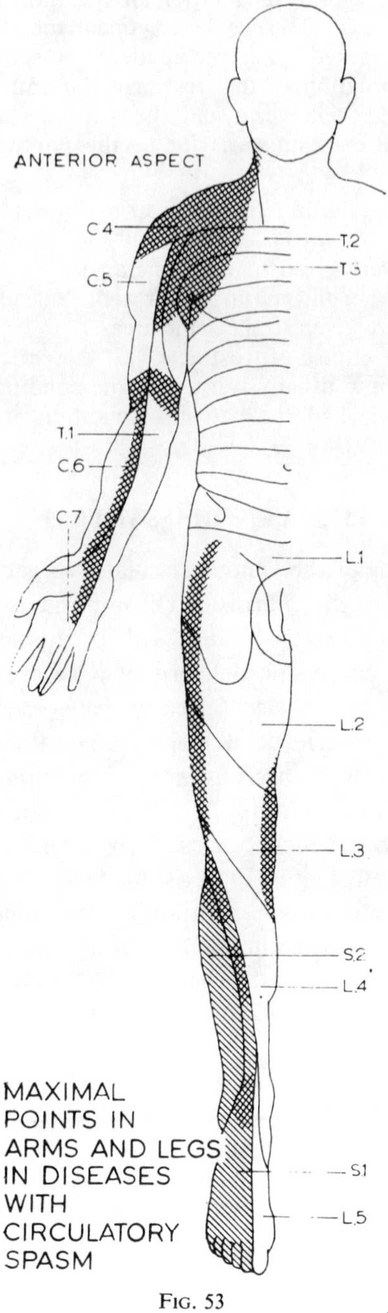
ANTERIOR ASPECT
C4
T.2
T.3
C.5
T.1
C.6
C.7
L.1
L.2
L.3
S.2
L.4
S.1
L.5
MAXIMAL POINTS IN ARMS AND LEGS IN DISEASES WITH CIRCULATORY SPASM

FIG. 53

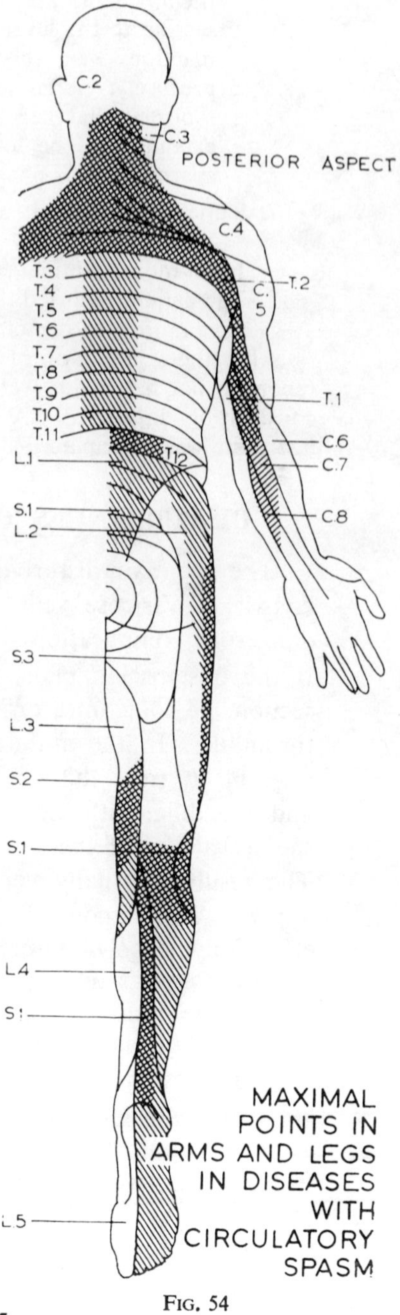
C2
C.3
POSTERIOR ASPECT
C.4
T.2
C. 5
T.3
T.4
T.5
T.6
T.7
T.8
T.9
T.10
T.11
T12
T.1
C.6
C.7
C.8
L.1
S.1
L.2
S.3
L.3
S.2
S.1
L.4
S1
L.5
MAXIMAL POINTS IN ARMS AND LEGS IN DISEASES WITH CIRCULATORY SPASM

FIG. 54

them. Same areas treated, with addition of the thoracic section to the level of C.7. During the treatment the skin reaction was very marked and the patient perspired profusely. After termination of the treatment the patient reported that her hands felt warm and the warm feeling extended in the lower extremities as far as the popliteal space.

7. Same areas treated, with addition of the anterior border of trapezius.

Four more treatments were given to the same areas.

12. The patient reported that her fingers no longer went "dead."

Five more treatments were given to the same areas.

After the termination of the course of treatment (17) the patient reported that her hands were now usually warm and the condition considerably improved. A review of the patient's condition at a later date was anticipated.

DISTURBANCES OF THE VENOUS SYSTEM

The two main disturbances of the venous circulatory system consist of varicose veins and thrombosis. Thrombosis is a dangerous complication sometimes associated with pregnancy. If the obstetrician plans to carry out delivery by Caesarean section, he sometimes orders massage in order to disperse the thrombus. In the author's experience it is perfectly safe to attempt to treat this condition if carefully applied effleurage and kneading, with the limbs in elevation, is applied, avoiding the actual site of the thrombus which can easily by palpated. The result is usually very satisfactory. It is inadvisable to apply C.T.M. under these conditions because of the reflex effect on the pelvic viscera. Present knowledge about uterine function is too inadequate to exclude the possibility of a miscarriage induced reflexly. The author personally would therefore not take the risk.

Varicose veins are dilated veins which have rendered the valves incompetent. It is now generally accepted that individuals are constitutionally predisposed to this condition and it is thought to result from venous stasis rather than from increased venous pressure. As mentioned under Blood Vessels, the walls of vessels are nourished from two main sources, one being the vasa vasorum which carry oxygenated blood into the wall from outside sources and the other being the supply to the walls derived from the blood carried by the vessels. Veins carry deoxygenated blood, and the health of the venous walls therefore depends primarily on the efficiency of the vasa vasorum. The chief manifestations of chronic venous insufficiency are in the skin and subcutaneous tissue. As a result of stasis the venous blood has a low content of oxygen and a high content of carbon dioxide and other products of metabolism. The nutrition of the tissues is impaired and oedema and necrosis may result. Ulceration of a limb with venous stasis may occur at the site of a local thrombosis of small superficial veins, or it may follow trauma with broken skin. The healing power of the poorly nourished tissues is affected and trauma may not be followed by repair. Hence ulceration is a common complication of chronic venous insufficiency (Anning, 1949). The treatment of this condition by a combination of Bisgaard massage and ointment prescribed by the physician is usually very effective. There are, however, cases which are resistant to this treatment and it is for this reason that the treatment by C.T.M. is outlined below. C.T.M. will not only affect the peripheral capillary circulation but will probably also have a reflex effect on the vasa vasorum and so contribute to the health of the venous vessels. The advantage in these cases is the fact that the massage will not be carried out in the periphery over skin which easily breaks down under manipulation, but will be applied to the appropriate segments in the back.

Outline of investigation and treatment

In all cases of venous-lymphatic stasis the tissue in the back over the lumbar region, and particularly below the iliac crest, will appear to be drawn in and show increased tension, while the area over the great trochanter of the femur appears swollen. Tension over the ilio-tibial tract is increased, and this area may be sensitive to palpation. The colour of the skin over the extremity and over the pelvic region may appear bluish. In

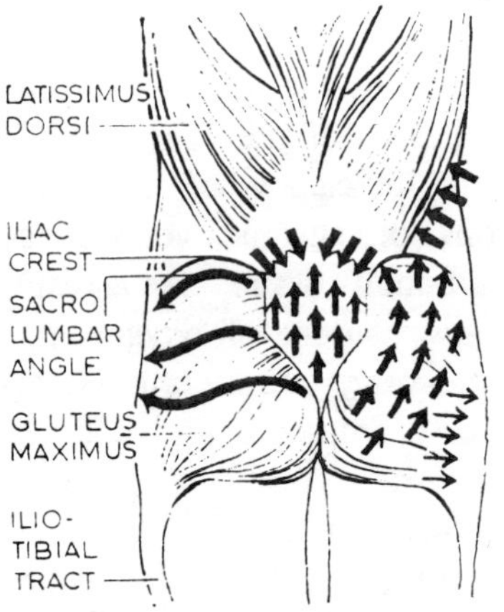

STROKES OVER SACRAL AND GLUTEAL REGION IN VENOUS-LYMPHATIC DISTURBANCE

Fig. 55

most cases a satisfactory result may already be obtained during the treatment of the basic section and the upper part of the thigh and it will not be necessary to pass farther into the periphery. In some resistant cases with organized lymph stasis it may be necessary to treat the lower leg. This will produce a dilatation of blood capillaries with increased permeability. which will facilitate colloid return.

It is advisable to carry out the treatment in the forward lying, lying or side lying position. It is essential, particularly in the early treatments, to work with very short strokes carried through the tissues very slowly because of the existing fluid stasis and increased tension. The irritation may be the result of strokes carried out too quickly or strokes being forced through tense tissue.

The back treatment should be carried to the level of T.10, including the latissimus dorsi area. Concentrated treatment of the pelvic and sacral areas is important, especially the sacro-lumbar angle. The sacral area tension will be relieved by very short lifting strokes passing upwards over the posterior aspect of the sacrum.

The whole of the buttock area should be treated in a similar way, leading the short strokes at right angles to the direction of fibres of gluteus maximus. When the tension in this area decreases, the short strokes can be followed by longer strokes in the direction parallel to the iliac crest, carrying them forward as far as possible to the groin. If the great saphenous vein is particularly affected, the sartorius border should be treated (Fig. 34). These strokes usually produce a very intensive cutting sensation and must therefore be carried out at little depth and very slowly.

If lymphatic stasis of the lower leg is a predominant symptom special attention should be paid to the treatment of the posterior border of the ilio-tibial tract and, on the medial side, the area round the adductor hiatus. Great care should be taken.

The treatment for circulatory stasis should be carried out initially several times a week, gradually decreasing the frequency. After the first few treatments patients usually report beneficial results as related to the ability to stand for longer periods without severe discomfort, and the colour of the leg shows improvement. It is, however, beneficial if the patient can avoid long standing, but carry out walks of increasing length. In very chronic conditions, particularly on a constitutional basis, a few treatment sessions should be repeated once a year, preferably before the beginning of the warm weather.

It must be realised that lower costal and abdominal breathing plays an important part in venous return. Very little of the impetus produced during the systolic and diastolic phase of the cardiac contraction is carried into the venous part of the circulatory system. The pumping action of muscles and the action of the diaphragm are therefore of vital importance for venous return in the lower limb. During the inspiratory phase the dome of the diaphragm flattens. This causes a decrease in pressure in the chest cavity and an increase inpressure in the abdominal cavity which becomes particularly effective on the thinner walled vessels such as the inferior vena cava. This pressure change produces the effect of a pressure pump on the abdominal part of this vessel and the effect of a suction pump on the thoracic part. The outer wall of the vessel blends with the central tendon of the diaphragm and during the flattening phase of the muscle will increase the lumen of the main returning vessel. As previously mentioned relaxation of the abdominal wall in circulatory conditions should be achieved by raising the head and shoulders by means of a soft pillow.

Case History: 19.12.1980

Female, aged 75: Housewife

The patient had from the age of 20 a tendency to varicose veins and very poor circulation, hands and feet cold even in the Summer. The condition was aggravated during pregnancy 40 years ago. At present a fairly extensive ulcer exists above the left medical malleolus, which has been treated by the G.P. during the last five weeks with various dressings, including Quinaband and bandaging to knee level. A great deal of pain during day and night causes sleep disturbance.

Back Inspection: Venous zone left + +, right +
Liver zone + (cannot eat eggs and fat)

Treatment: 1) Forward lying. Basic section, buttocks, hamstring area. Only short strokes used. Lying - both legs to popliteal space. Breathing exercises taught.
On departure still painful.

2) 3 days later: Pain free during night and day, yesterday pain in the morning. As last time.

3) 29.12.1980 Christmas interfered with treatment. Patient much more cheerful, no throbbing pain, toes less blue. C.T.M. to same areas

4) 5.1.1981 Yesterday for the first time slight stabbing pain over ulcerated area which is healing

Five more treatments were given at weekly intervals with C.T.M., patient practises breathing exercises and circulatory exercises.

16.2.1981 Ulcer now completely healed, patient only wears Tubigrip bandage. Treatment as before plus latissimus dorsi and upper arms to elbow.

23.2.1981 Patient feels very well
Treatment with C.T.M.: Basic section, Back to T7, Latissimus Dorsi, scapula, two upper arms, stress biceps, hamstring area to popliteal space, 2 thighs

On departure patient feels very well and glowing!
No further trouble up to end of 1983.

P.S. The author has lately been able to obtain complete healing and restoration of healthy skin in a chronic case of ulceration in the lower leg, aggravated by a complicated fracture into the hip joint due to a motor accident. Treatment consisted of C.T.M. and a modified form of Buerger's exercises, leaving out the dependent phase.

LYMPHATIC LESIONS

These may manifest themselves in two main directions. In

certain patients the lymphatics are more prone to be influenced by heat and gravity than in others, without the presence of heart disease. This manifests itself particularly in the ankle region, on the dorsum of the foot and along the Tendo-achilles. These areas show swelling in situations such as long air journeys, bus rides or car journeys or long periods of standing or sitting. In many cases this swelling disappears after a night's rest but in a number of patients the situation does not resolve itself completely and gradually the fluid becomes organised in the subcutaneous tissues and hardens. This reduces joint mobility in the affected areas and causes the patient discomfort. Elevation helps in the beginning but gradually becomes less effective.

The second group of patients show similar symptoms, but the swelling is more pronounced, the skin becomes glossy and the swelling is often painful. These patients are diagnosed as suffering from Sudeck's Atrophy which is now considered to be of neurogenic origin by most authorities. It is a complication which appears fairly suddenly and unexpectedy in association with injuries, particularly fractures in the upper or lower limb. It is more frequent in the upper limb, the reason for it is unknown. In desperate cases sympathectomy of the ganglia in the area is performed, usually with no lasting effect. The puzzling factor is that the complication usually appears 6-8 weeks after the original trauma which in itself has been resolved and successfully treated. I have treated three patients with this complication in the upper limb, in two cases the swelling was in the hand, in one case in the elbow region. This points to the fact that the pathology is associated with areas of extensive vascular anastomosis. In all three cases C.T.M. was applied and successful.

As I was walking on virgin ground and no other treatment had been successful, I had to reason out the rationale of the treatment. I considered that it was essential to encourage absorption by freeing more centrally situated channels. This would increase the effectiveness of the respiratory and muscular pump.

The Back Inspection was carried out in sitting and showed flattened areas over the anterior and posterior surfaces of deltoid and a very tight latissimus dorsi fascia. Two of the patients had suffered a fracture into the head of the humerus, one into the humeral shaft, caused by a fall on the shoulder.

I should like to summarize the treatment of one shoulder patient who was specially co-operative because he was a keen fisherman and had arranged a fishing holiday to take place in two months' time. At the beginning of the treatment he had shoulder movement to shoulder level.

C.T.M. treatment in forward lying: Short strokes to the Basic section, continued after two treatments to T7, latissimus dorsi fascia, *both* scapulae, with short strokes only. At the third treatment the patient was placed additionally into the lying position with the whole arm supported on pillows in elevation. C.T.M. short strokes to the clavicular and deltoid and axillary areas, carefully progressing on further sessions to the elbow region. More than in any other condition, the principle must be observed that no manipulation or stroke is painful to the patient. The affected hand must not be touched until the swelling has almost completely disappeared and no discomfort is present. With the patient in lying with head and shoulders elevated—abdominal and lower costal breathing is taught for frequent practise at home. Exercises for the upper limb, supported in the elevated position, should at first be restricted to shoulder movements, assisted by the sound limb, followed by elbow movements to the limit of the pain free range. All functional hand movements should never be carried beyond the limit of discomfort. The patient could arrange to be driven to his office and therefore carry out his work as managing director of a woolen mill.

I have treated a number of patients with lower limb oedema, not diagnosed as Sudeck's Atrophy, on similar lines, all were greatly improved and restriction to lower limb mobility prevented.

SCARS

Scars caused by burns can be considerably improved by improving the circulation either to the affected limb or the head if the scars have occurred in the face. In one case it was possible to improve the movement range in a patient's hand where severe contractures had occurred after skin grafting. The post-operative treatment at the time of the grafting had been neglected due to various uncontrollable circumstances. The overall extension in the hand was measured from the heel of the hand to the finger-tips. An increase of extension from $1\frac{3}{8}$ to $2\frac{1}{2}$ inches was possible. The number of treatments given was forty-nine.

In another patient with severe bitumen burns C.T.M. was given prior to skin grafting. Almost complete healing of the wounds was achieved and the movement range improved. The number of treatments was sixty-nine.

Treatment

This again starts with the basic section and should progress quickly into the affected segments. It must be remembered that all injuries in the head or face region will produce tension alteration between the scapulae. It is therefore important to concentrate the back treatment in that area, especially as these patients very often suffer from headaches which respond very badly to drugs.

The circulation round the individual scar should be improved by short lifting strokes towards the centre of the scar.

CHAPTER XI

Reflex Symptoms within the Metamer

THIS chapter attempts to discuss some alterations in *tissues of the body surface* caused by *pathological organic conditions* and the appearance of symptomatic organic dysfunction due to *pathological conditions in other tissues* of the same segmental supply. One of the earliest suggestions of widespread reaction in the various tissues depending for their innervation on the original segmental nerve centre came from the English neurologist, Head, and the surface alterations described by Head are now known in the literature as Head's zones. Later English authors, such as Mennell (1945), Cyriax (1950) and Schleyer-Saunders (1955), to mention only a few, have discussed the implications of these early findings, while some of these early discoveries have become universally accepted in the medical literature (*e.g.* altered surface tension in the abdomen in acute appendicitis). Many continental investigators, some of whom will be mentioned later, have provided an extensive literature to prove that (*a*) pathological conditions of organs cause reflexly pathological symptoms in the skin and the connective tissue element of the body surface, in the muscles, blood vessels and nerves, probably also in the bones if they depend for their innervation on the same segmental nerve supply; (*b*) pathological conditions of the tissues of the body surface including the skin and its connective tissue element, muscles and bones will eventually cause pathological dysfunction of organs within the same segmental nerve supply; (*c*) therapeutic agents applied to the surface tissues of the segment will influence beneficially the pathological condition of the affected organs within the segment.

It would be beyond the scope of this book to discuss the implications of pathological conditions mentioned under (*b*).

Some of the continental authors quoted below may help to illustrate the statements made under (*a*) and (*c*).

It is a universally recognized factor that in the presence of angina pectoris, spontaneous pain and pain caused by touch of the left pectoral region arises in that region, radiating into the left arm. Wernoe (1925), Knotz (1927), Kayser-Petersen (1930) and others reported changes in segmental tissues associated with diseases of the respiratory system. Dittmar (1943) and Rouanet (1946) reported circulatory changes in the capillaries of segments sharing the same nerve supply with pathologically affected organs. Opperman (1949) reported dermographic changes within the skin segments associated with the pathology of abdominal organs.

Kohlrausch (1953) discussed extensively the peripheral changes associated with organic disturbances as well as the therapeutic effect of peripheral application of massage and exercises on pathologically affected organs. Nonnenbruch and Gross (1952) observed organic disturbances, neuralgia, lumbago, migraine, arthropathies due to circulatory disturbances in the presence of scar tissue or chronic inflammatory changes in various parts of the body. They consider that these organic disturbances follow vascular channels over arterio-arterial reflexes. These reflexes seem to represent an explanation of many pathological disturbances which cannot be explained as reflex symptoms within the segmental distribution. According to these authors, therapeutic applications should be applied following the principles which were responsible for the disturbance, *i.e.* to the focus of the disturbance. This will explain in some cases the removal of peripheral symptoms through C.T.M. in the back, although the back segments treated do not correspond to the dermatome area in the periphery. The following chapter discusses the treatment of organic disturbances by C.T.M. The information is largely taken from German sources but the author has been able to confirm in a number of cases the beneficial effect of the treatment. The results have been obtained chiefly with patients who were treated for conditions such as rheumatism or backache of unknown origin, and the relief of symptoms such as asthma or constipation was incidental. The information contained in the publications by Niebauer and al. (1972, 1977) will shed further light on the relationship between surface tissues and organs. Future experience under the guidance of the medical profession and representatives of allied sciences should prove very valuable.

HEART DISEASES

Cardiac symptoms may be due to a variety of causes. All symptoms of cardiac insufficiency are profoundly disturbing to the patient even if these symptoms are not caused by organic disease. Connective tissue massage carried out in very close co-operation with the medical practitioner will in most cases provide great relief to the patient and allow return to a more normal kind of life. In functional types of abnormal heart function the massage must be combined with a carefully graded scheme of exercises. Associated symptoms with all types of cardiac disease, such as stiff neck, shoulder and arm pains, can in most cases be greatly relieved by C.T.M. and in many cases the patient cán become symptom-free for long periods. In all cases it is essential that the physiotherapist should be well-informed and conversant with the patient's history, particularly the severity of the organic disease in such cases as coronary thrombosis or cardiac stenosis.

Zones affected

IN THE BACK. The areas affected may reach from C.3 to T.9. Some of these areas are painful on movement. This applies particularly to the junction of neck and shoulder over the anterior margin of trapezius and the shoulder joint area over the posterior fibres of deltoid. The costal areas over the segments 2 to 4 and 9 to 10 are often drawn in, while the tissue towards the axillary margin of the same segments appears swollen with a sharp drawn-in border over latissimus dorsi. All these changes are present on the left side of the thorax, but some tissue changes may be observed over the right liver area, particularly if the portal circulation is affected.

IN FRONT. The changes can be observed in the same segments as in the back. The intercostal spaces over T.2 and T.6 to T.7 may be painful on pressure. The tissues along the inferior margin of the clavicle, over the origin of sternomastoid and the lateral part of pectoralis major appear drawn in, while the tissues over the left lateral margin of the sternum appear

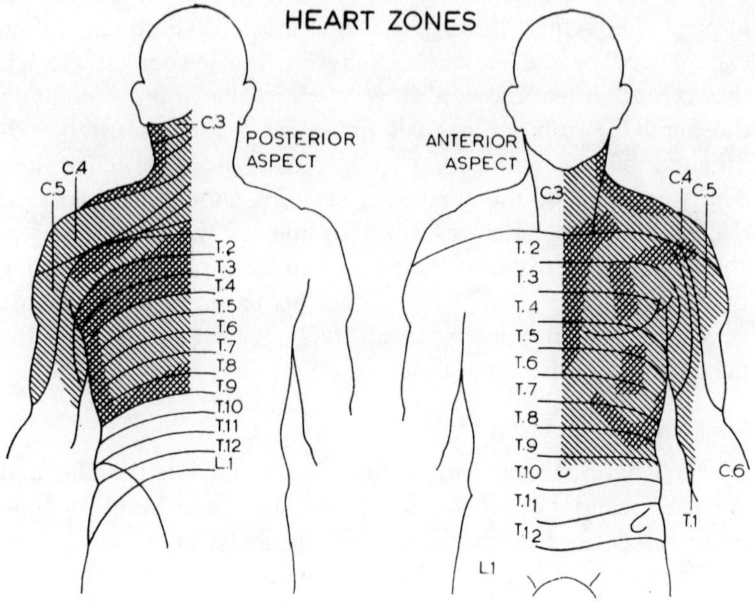

FIG. 56

swollen. Radiating pains are often mentioned by the patient over the anterior part of deltoid and along the medial aspect of the arm.

Treatment

As far as possible the treatment should be carried out in the sitting position and the patient must have a short rest period after the treatment. The early treatment sessions should not exceed twenty minutes and should be repeated two or three times a week. For approximately two weeks only the basic section should be included in the treatment, the patient's satisfactory progress determining the inclusion of thoracic and cervical segments. The latissimus dorsi area should be treated before encroaching on the more medially situated parts of the back. No strokes over pectoralis major should be applied until the tension areas over the back have improved considerably. From the beginning, shallow, superficial strokes along the clavicle and strokes along the subcostal margin should be applied frequently during the treatment. These are often experienced by the patient as relieving the tension in the left thorax and often provoke a very noticeable improvement in the depth of respiration. All treatment sessions must be terminated by the application of subcostal and pelvic strokes. The frequency of the treatment sessions should gradually be decreased. The anterior aspect of the left intercostal spaces should only be treated if the patient still complains of a feeling of tension. The attempt to relieve this tension must be made very carefully and interspersed freely with treatment of the pelvic and subcostal margins.

Summary of treatment

First basic section only, progressing to include thoracic and cervical sections but excluding the left side until definite improvement has taken place. Left clavicular area.

Treatment of left side of thorax posteriorly and progression to right anterior aspect of pectoral region.

Throughout the treatment period emphasis is laid on the left subcostal margin. Left pectoral region only treated if necessary.

RESPIRATORY CONDITIONS

The conditions which benefit by the application of C.T.M., according to the German authors and the author's own experience, are chronic bronchitis and the frequently associated bronchiectasis and asthma, especially in resistant cases. In all these conditions the treatment must be combined with the appropriate breathing exercises and the teaching of relaxation.

In bronchiectasis the patient must also be taught the drainage positions for the affected lobes for regular home practice. In all conditions of unilateral pathology, *e.g.* bronchiectasis, the connective tissue zones may be present or more pronounced on the affected side only. Should a cardiac involvement aggravate the respiratory pathology, additional heart zones may be present and the treatment will have to be progressed carefully. Particular tension areas are present in the shoulder and neck regions which must, however, not be treated until the tension in the more caudally situated areas has been relieved. The patient's report relating to the sensation following the massage stroke is particularly important. Dull pressure report instead of a clear cutting sensation is indicative of unrelieved tension in lower segments. The treatment should therefore immediately return to the treatment of these areas. The areas of C.7 and the external occipital protuberance very often show swellings which disappear when the tension in the lower segments has been relieved. Tension in the anterior aspect of the thorax will improve during the treatment of the posterior aspect but will require careful attention during the later phases of treatment. During the early treatment sessions it may be difficult to obtain the cutting reaction, and no progression must be attempted until this has been achieved in the basic section. The stimulation of the appropriate trigger points in the various sections will, in most cases, eventually be successful in obtaining the desired reflex reaction.

Zones affected

IN THE BACK. The zones affected reach from C.3 to C.8 and T.1 to T.9; in asthma they may include the whole back as far down as L.5. Tension areas are present on either side of the vertebral column, especially between the scapulae and on either side of the external occipital protuberance, the areas over the posterior part of deltoid and over the sternoclavicular joint. In bronchitic conditions the lower costal margin and the lateral margin of latissimus dorsi may also show increased tension; in asthma these tension areas are always present.

Asthma may show additional tension areas over the iliac crests.

IN FRONT. The zones affected and showing increased tension are in particular the areas of attachment of sternomastoid and the borders of this muscle, the areas along the lateral borders of the sternum over the chondrosternal articulations, the

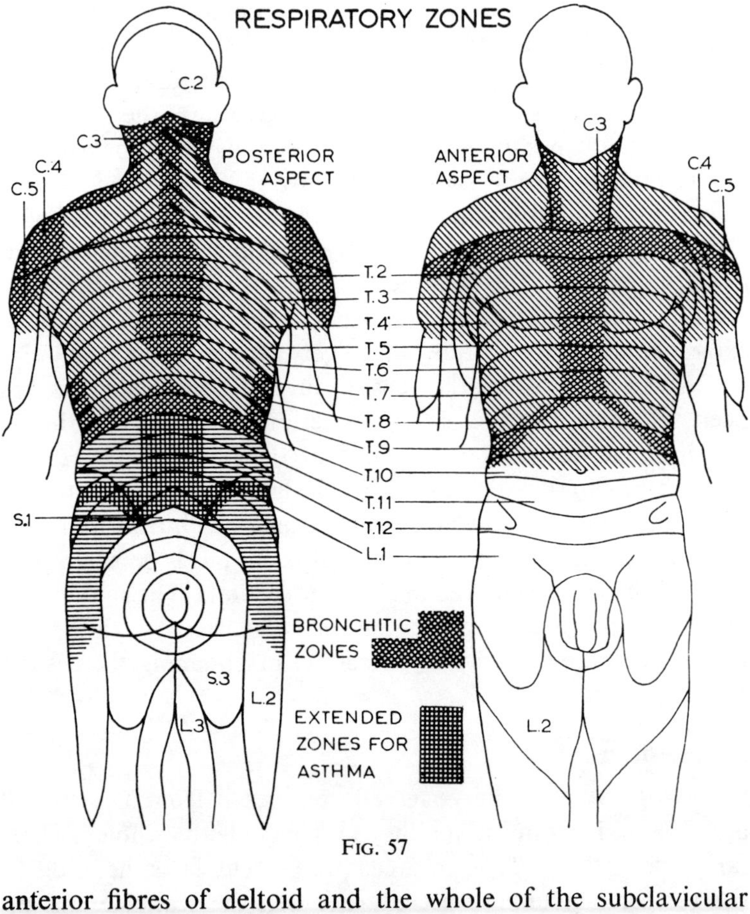

FIG. 57

anterior fibres of deltoid and the whole of the subclavicular margin. In asthmatic patients the axillary portions of latissimus dorsi and pectoralis major are often particularly tense in addition to the anterior portion of the subcostal margin.

Treatment

Where possible the back should be treated in sitting or forward lean sitting against pillows. Clear reactions in the basic section are essential and particular attention should be paid to the angle between the vertebral column and the last rib, which should be treated with short, fan-like lifting strokes before an attempt is made to treat the intercostal spaces. Next follows the latissimus dorsi margin and then the whole thoracic and scapular regions. The area between the scapulae should be treated in the way used for headache treatment before an attempt is made to encroach on the cervical segments. Stretching of the posterior wall of the axilla often proves useful. At this point the patient usually already finds diaphragmatic breathing easier. Should difficulty still exist, treatment of the anterior abdominal wall in lying may bring relief. Strokes used pass over the iliac crest down to the symphysis pubis, starting lateral to the anterior superior iliac spine on both sides. Treatment of the lateral margin of rectus abdominis with short lifting strokes, carefully and not too deeply applied, introduce the treatment of the anterior subcostal margin. This again is treated with short lifting strokes, avoiding the epigastric angle. If clear reactions are obtained the treatment is continued into the cervical region. Special attention is paid to the angle formed by the spine of the scapula and the clavicle, the anterior border of trapezius and the occipital curved line. Progressing, the anterior aspect of the thorax can now be treated, including the clavicle and sterno-mastoid. Finally an attempt is made to ease the tension over the area of the sternum by passing short shallow strokes, gradually increasing in depth, in the intercostal spaces, starting approximately two inches lateral to the sternum. These areas are often very sensitive. After favourable response the strokes can be lengthened to cover the lower three to four intercostal spaces in their whole length. The treatment of these areas should be frequently interspersed with iliac crest strokes, which should also terminate every treatment.

Summary of treatment

Sitting or forward lean sitting, basic section with emphasis on the angle between lowest rib and vertebral column, latissimus dorsi, thoracic section with emphasis on the area between the scapulae, axillary stretching. In lying, pelvic margin, lateral margin of rectus abdominis, subcostal margin. Progression to cervical section with emphasis on angle between scapular spine and clavicle, occipital curved line. Anteriorly clavicle, intercostal spaces. Treatment interspersed freely with iliac crest and subcostal strokes and flat handed strokes anteriorly over clavicular area which also must terminate every treatment. Breathing training essential in all conditions.

DISORDERS OF THE DIGESTIVE SYSTEM

This group comprises a great variety of conditions which may benefit from C.T.M. These include diseases of the stomach, the intestinal tract and the portal system. It seems unnecessary to mention that no chartered physiotherapist will undertake the treatment of patients without the order of a medical practitioner. It is, however, important to mention that a number of these conditions may be in the chronic stage when treatment is started and may pass for various reasons into an acute phase again. It is therefore particularly important to watch the progress of the patient and report any new symptoms to the doctor immediately in order to avoid disastrous results in conditions such as gastric or duodenal ulcer, which may suddenly flare up again. The physiotherapist must also strictly abstain from giving any advice with regard to diet or homely remedies such as milk of magnesia, etc., without consulting the physician. It should, however, be remembered that the additional teaching of breathing exercises in all digestive disorders can only benefit the patient. The increased oxygen supply will benefit all metabolic processes, while the rhythmic descent and elevation of the diaphragm will exert an alternate pressure and relaxation on organs such as the stomach and the liver, and assist their natural function.

STOMACH

The treatment may prove beneficial in cases of chronic

gastritis or gastric ulcer or after an acute attack has subsided while symptoms in the back and part of the abdominal wall are still present. It is the treatment of choice in all cases of functional disturbance without pathological background. This applies to cases of increased general tension which may be due to psychological disturbances.

Zones affected

The segments affected may reach from C.3 to C.8 and T.5 to T.9 on the left side of the body but may extend in the thoracic section into the right side if the liver participates in the functional disturbance.

IN THE BACK. The areas particularly increased in tension can be found lateral to the vertebral column in the thoracic segments 7 and 8, over the inferior angle of the left scapula in segment 5 and an area in the infraspinous fossa of the scapula in its lateral part just below the scapular spine. This point is almost invariably painful on palpation and may also give discomfort on deep breathing. It should be avoided in the early treatment sessions and no attempt should be made to relieve the tension until all other tension areas have cleared up. It is a point which will flare up whenever there is a minor flare-up in the patient's condition. An inconstant painful tension area may also be found in the cervical segment 3 and 4 over the anterior margin of the left trapezius.

IN FRONT. Two specially affected areas may be noted in the thoracic segments 7 and 8 in mid-clavicular line and over the left rectus abdominis. In the neck, tension may be present over the angle formed by sternomastoid and the clavicle.

Treatment

The treatment should be carried out in the sitting or forward lean sitting position and begun with the basic section which almost invariably shows general increased tissue tension. At this stage particular attention should be paid to the treatment of the lower costal margin on the left side. The skin reaction at first is often very bright red and the stroke areas show wheal formation. It is important to terminate every treatment with strokes which are carried forward over the anterior superior iliac spines and the iliac crest in order to avoid change of tension into the anterior tissue areas. As soon as the tension in the basic section and the costal margin is reduced the strokes are progressed posteriorly into the thoracic region but avoiding the scapulae. The intercostal spaces should first be approached with short lifting strokes before an attempt is made to ease

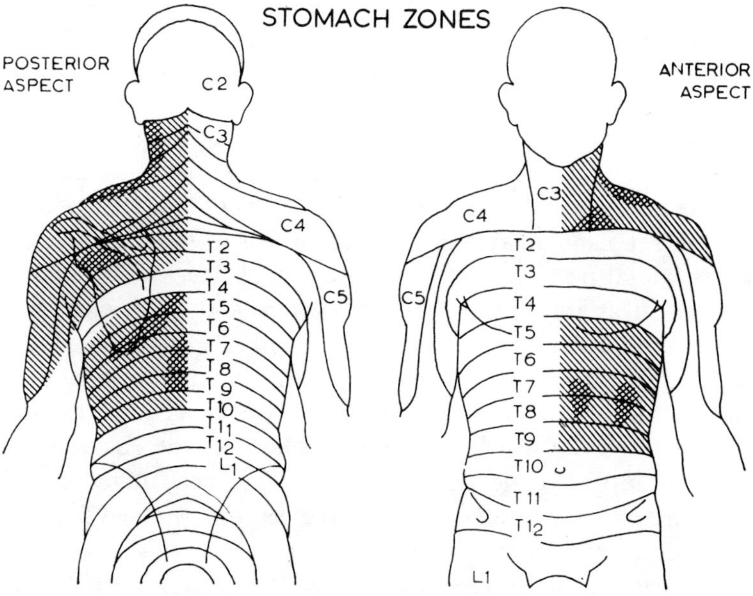

FIG. 58

the tension with long strokes passing along the spaces from lateral to medial. The treatment of the scapulae should not be attempted until the tension over the left inferior scapular angle has been reduced. Should pain over the maximal point below the left scapular spine still be present this point must be avoided until the tension in the whole infraspinous fossa has been normalized. It will not be necessary in many cases to treat the anterior aspect of the thorax as the tension areas will have disappeared during the back treatment. Should final palpation still reveal anterior tension areas these should be treated in the lying position, starting with the lower costal margin and intercostal spaces with short lifting strokes which are followed by longer strokes in the direction of the ribs from lateral to medial. It is advisable to avoid at first the maximal point areas, gradually encroaching on them. Every treatment must be terminated with strokes covering the iliac crest, including the anterior superior iliac spine.

The frequency of treatments should gradually be reduced, starting with two to three per week to one a week and finally every other week. This will give the necessary information that the patient is symptom-free and can lead a normal life.

Summary of treatment

First basic section in sitting or forward lean sitting with emphasis on left costal margin. Progression to thoracic section with exclusion of scapulae. After successful release of tension over inferior scapular angle progression to scapulae with careful approach to maximal point below scapular spine. If necessary final treatment over anterior thoracic aspect in lying. Every treatment to be terminated with strokes over the iliac crest.

INTESTINAL TRACT

The treatment may prove beneficial after the subsidence of acute inflammatory conditions of the small intestine, such as duodenal ulcers, enteritis and colitis which continue to leave abnormal tension areas in the anterior and posterior walls of the abdominal cavity. It is particularly useful in intestinal disturbances due to general psychological tension, and proves successful in all cases of chronic constipation both of the atonic and the spastic types. As previously stressed the treatment is never given without medical advice and may therefore only represent part of the general treatment of this distressing condition which always affects the general health due to lack of efficient elimination of waste products. In the atonic type it will probably be associated with general and specific exercises to the abdominal muscles; in the spastic type, which is often due to neurasthenia, it will be combined with the teaching of relaxation. In both types breathing exercises will prove valuable due to the rhythmic descent and elevation of the diaphragm producing alternate pressure and relaxation on the abdominal content and due to the relief of abdominal circulatory stasis. The doctor will have investigated dietetic and hygienic errors in the life of the patient and the physiotherapist must during treatment time help to impress on the patient the importance of carrying out the doctor's advice. It is most important for the patient to realize that his active co-operation is most essential as many of these patients have become accustomed to outside help and may approach the new treatment in the same spirit.

During the investigation by palpation and for mobility of superficial tissues on deep tissues, general increase in tension can usually be found in all lumbar and lower thoracic segments; sometimes this is also present in the sacral areas, especially in all cases of spastic constipation. In spastic constipation it is very important to concentrate on the area between the ischial tuberosity and the great trochanter. For effective treatment it is sometimes advisable to treat the patient in the side-lying position, which must be made comfortable with the support of pillows in front. Patients suffering from spastic constipation sometimes complain of discomfort in the peripheral distribution of lumbar segments along the upper and inner part of the thigh. This discomfort disappears when the tension in the posterior distribution has been relieved and in most cases need not be treated specially. The treatment of the ilio-lumbar angle is particularly important and must be started very carefully as it frequently proves very painful. During treatment, back tension is often transferred to the front, and no treatment should be terminated before the anterior parts of the iliac crest and the areas of the anterior superior iliac spine have finally been treated in the lying position by deep stroking along the crest and round the spine.

Zones affected

The segments affected may reach from T.6 to S.2 with radiating zones into the cervical segments 3 to 5.

IN THE BACK. *Duodenum.* The right thoracic region T.6 to T.10 with increased tension over T.8 to T.9.

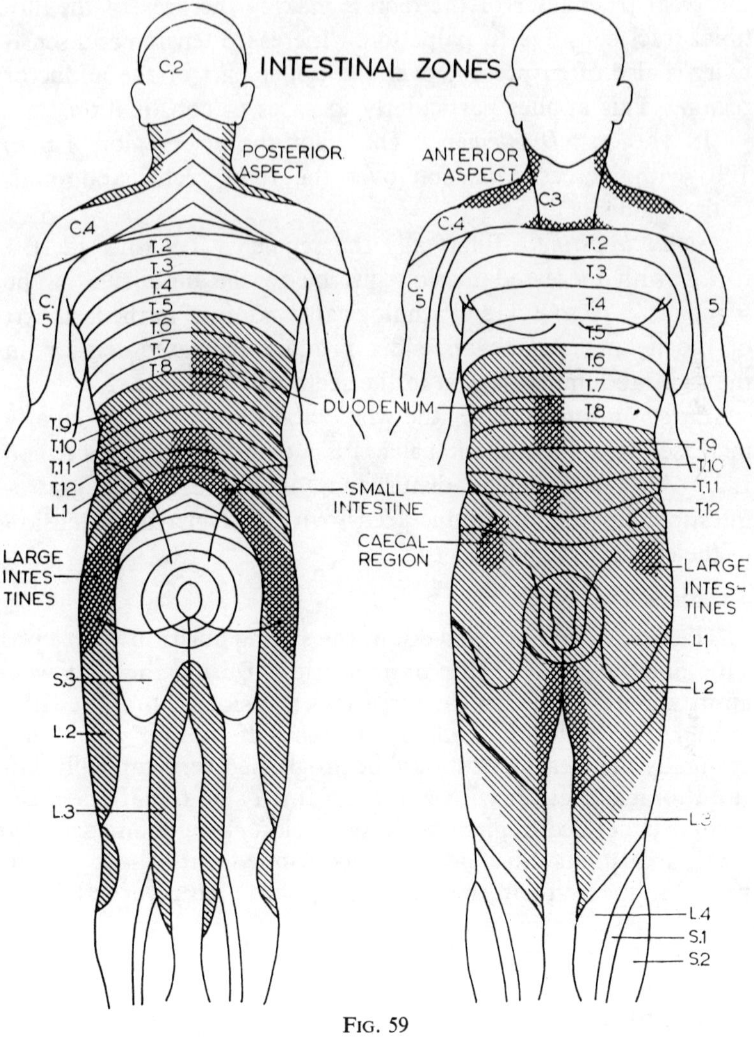

FIG. 59

Small intestine. On both sides of the vertebral column T.9 to T.12 and L.1 to L.5 with increased tension over L.3 to L.4 in all cases where diarrhoea is the main symptom.

Large intestine. On both sides of the vertebral column in the segments T.12, L.1 to L.5 and S.1 with increased tension on both sides over the middle one-third of the sacrum, radiating towards the great trochanter of the femur, making the area of the ilio-tibial tract sensitive to palpation. Increased tension and sensitivity is also often present over the upper part of the adductor region. This applies particularly to cases of constipation.

IN FRONT. *Duodenum.* The right thoracic region T.6 to T.10 with increased tension over the right rectus abdominis in the segments 8 to 9.

Small intestine. Bilaterally the segments T.9 to T.12, L.1 to L.5 with increased tension just below the umbilicus in the segments T.10 to T.11. Pathological conditions in the last part of the ileum and the appendix produce increased tension in the right abdominal region in the segments T.12 to L.2.

Large intestine. Over the whole abdomen with particularly increased tension in the left iliac fossa over the segments L.1 to L.2. Any pathological disturbance anywhere in the gastro-intestinal tract may produce sensitivity and increased tension in the cervical segments 3 to 5.

Treatment

The treatment is carried out in the sitting position where possible and begun with the basic section. During the first week approximately three to four treatment sessions should be fitted in and followed every time by at least half an hour's rest. Only gradually the treatment should be progressed very carefully into the thoracic section with emphasis finally on the affected segments. If cervical segments show tension changes and sensitive areas, treatment must not be discontinued until these changes have disappeared and the patient's appetite has returned.

CONSTIPATION

Treatment

The treatment should be started in the sitting position with special emphasis on the sacral area and the angle between lumbar spine and posterior superior iliac spine. Treatment of the iliac crest and the anterior superior iliac spine will soon produce improvement in the anterior abdominal tension. During the first treatment the patient should be placed in the lying position in order to treat the great trochanter of the femur and the ilio-tibial tract. As soon as the abdominal tension has improved the thoracic sections should be treated, including careful treatment of the intercostal spaces.

The additional practice of breathing exercises proves beneficial both for atonic as well as for spastic constipation. In cases of atonic constipation simple exercises for all the abdominal muscles prove beneficial; in cases of spastic constipation the patient must be taught relaxation. In all cases it is important to ascertain that the patient is following the doctor's advice with regard to diet and general hygiene.

LIVER AND GALL-BLADDER

Connective tissue massage may prove helpful in cases of functional disturbances of the portal system and as treatment after inflammatory conditions have subsided. It will help reflexly to improve the circulation and this will improve functional activity. Additional teaching of breathing exercises, to be practised regularly by the patient, will enhance the effect. Patients often complain of sensitivity over the right abdominal and thoracic regions to slight amounts of pressure exerted by skirt or trouser fastenings. Pain is often present in the area between the right scapula and the thoracic spine and patients may complain of diffuse types of pain over the right shoulder region, radiating into the right arm, and sometimes even into the hand. These pains become particularly troublesome when the patient succumbs to the temptation of chocolate or eats fats of large molecular value, *e.g.*, pork. The patients frequently experience a feeling of general relief and buoyancy as soon as the lower costal margin is treated. This is understandable if one considers the importance of liver function on digestion and general body metabolism. Pain symptoms may flare up again over the maximal points due to general psychological upsets as long as the increased tension in the superficial tissues has not been removed. It is therefore advisable to decrease the frequency of treatments, starting with three treatments per week and gradually decreasing to one treatment per month.

In the author's experience the frequent use of comparatively heavy doses of antibiotics in sometimes trivial conditions represents a heavy burden on the liver. The reactive response of the liver may set up Tissue changes in the appropriate segments affecting superficial muscle and surface tissues. This causes loss of extensability in these tissues and affects the mobility of the thoracic spine. The result is pain on movement simulating an orthopaedic condition which does not respond to the usual therapeutic measures such as heat–traction and exercises. C.T.M. treatment removing the abnormal tension areas is very quickly rewarded with disappearance of pain and functional disturbance.

Manual investigation for changes in tissue tension and sensitivity shows that most thoracic segments from T.1 to T.10 are affected on the right side. Additional tension changes can be observed in the cervical segments 3 to 6, while the area over C.7 often shows a swelling. A point between the superior angle of the right scapula and the thoracic spine in the segments T.1 to T.3 is painful to touch and remains resistant to treatment for a long time. It is of particular importance as it is invariably present in all cases of liver involvement. It is often difficult to obtain a cutting reaction over this point and it must be excluded from treatment until the tension has been released in the lower, more caudally situated areas. When a reaction can be obtained the shoulder and arm symptoms start to improve rapidly. In many cases of troublesome arm symptoms a sensitive area can be detected over the right lateral margin of rectus abdominis at umbilical level. Touching of this point during treatment may produce a sudden spastic contraction of the muscle in addition to the pain. Treatment of the lower costal margin carried out anteriorly in the lying position during later treatment gives great relief to the patient.

Zones affected

The segments affected are chiefly on the right side from T.1 to T.10, radiating into the cervical segments 3 to 6.

IN THE BACK. Tension is particularly increased between the right scapula and the vertebral column at the level of T.4 to T.6 and over the inferior angle of the right scapula. The inferior costal margin appears to be drawn in and there is increased tension over the lateral margin of the right latissimus dorsi. A very sensitive area exists over the area between the right superior scapular angle and the thoracic spine at the level of T.1 to T.3. Tension is increased very frequently over the length of the lateral margin of trapezius, including the upper part of deltoid.

IN FRONT. The tension in the trapezius and deltoid areas is continued into the anterior aspect in the segments C3 to C6, and may also be present over the posterior margin of sterno-mastoid near its clavicular attachment. The drawn-in appearance of the subcostal margin is continued into the anterior aspect.

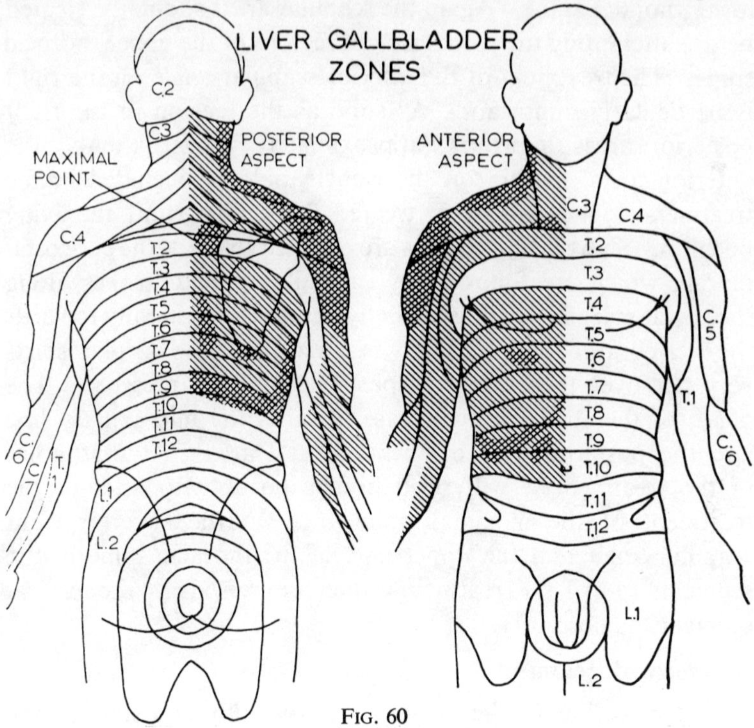

FIG. 60

Sensitive points are to be found in mid-clavicular line in the segments T6, T8 and T9 and over the right rectus abdominis. The latter point is particularly sensitive if the gall-bladder is involved.

Treatment

The treatment is started in the sitting position with the basic section, omitting, however, the ilio-sacral angle at first as it often proves too painful. The subcostal stroke can also usually only be carried out when the tension in the right paravertebral region has been improved by short lifting strokes passing into the angle between the last rib and vertebral column. The treatment of the thoracic section should be started over the lateral margin of latissimus dorsi and the tension in the right intercostal areas relieved by short lifting strokes passing in the intercostal spaces vertically from below upwards before attempting the treatment of the paravertebral regions in the lower thoracic spine. Again the scapular areas should be treated before attempting the paravertebral regions of the upper thoracic spine. The treatment of the inferior scapular angle on the right is particularly important. As soon as the tension in the right posterior areas improves (approximately six treatments) the anterior costal margin on the right should be included in the treatment. The patient is treated for this part in the lying position. Short lifting strokes are directed towards the subcostal margin which are followed by carefully applied strokes along the costal margin, starting medially and passing laterally towards the vertebral column. It is essential that the stroke starts very flat over the anterior aspect without any pressure. The depth of the stroke can increase towards the mid-axillary line and the posterior part of the subcostal area. At that point in the treatment it will probably be possible to attempt the treatment of the maximal point between the superior right scapular angle and the upper part of the thoracic spine in the segments T1 to T3. Treatment is then progressed into the cervical segments as necessary.

Summary of treatment

Basic section in the sitting position with omission of the ilio-sacral angle at first and treatment of costo-vertebral angle before treating subcostal margin. Progression to latissimus dorsi margin, intercostal areas, scapular areas with omission of maximal point in T1 to T3, then rest of thoracic region. Further progression to treatment of anterior subcostal margin in lying. Return to maximal point in the back and treatment of cervical region where necessary. Treatment terminated in lying by iliac crest strokes and subcostal strokes.

DISEASES OF THE URINARY SYSTEM

Conditions which benefit, according to the German authors and in a limited way according to the author's own experience, by the application of C.T.M. are inflammatory conditions of the kidney and the bladder after the acute attack is over, renal calculi which may have passed spontaneously or have been removed surgically, and enuresis nocturna. Inflammatory conditions of the urinary system may leave behind far-reaching connective tissue changes which give rise to widespread symptoms, not connected in the patient's mind with the original condition. Most of these conditions are very painful during the acute attack and therefore probably cause protective spasms in the neighbouring tissues. In enuresis nocturna the C.T.M. should produce improvement of the condition after four or five treatments unless an organic lesion is present (*e.g.* spina bifida) or the psychological component plays such an important part that the consultation of a psychiatrist is indicated.

KIDNEY DISEASES

The patient usually complains of backache, which may radiate into the abdominal region, and general stiffness. On investigation the sacral and pelvic regions show increased tension which is often continued downwards into the ilio-tibial tract and upwards into the latissimus dorsi fascia. The lower costal margin shows a drawn-in band in the segmental area of T.10; the area of the affected kidney often shows a sensitive swelling. A point between the scapula and the vertebral column in the segment T.4 is acutely sensitive to touch. The general stiffness is particularly noticed by the patient in the morning and may take some time to pass off. It may radiate into the neck and cause occipital headache. In all cases of unilateral pathology the changes are usually present on the affected side only.

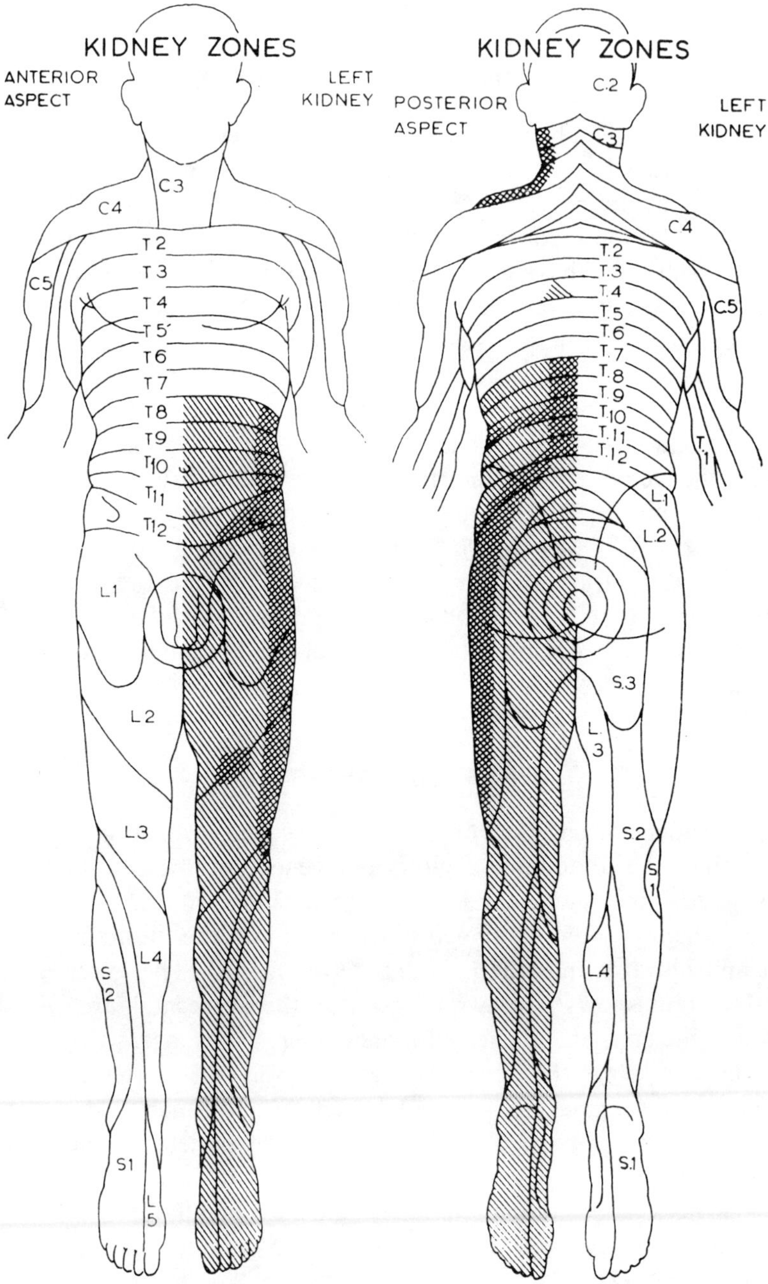
KIDNEY ZONES
ANTERIOR ASPECT
LEFT KIDNEY
C3
C4
T2
T3
C5
T4
T5
T6
T7
T8
T9
T10
T11
T12
L1
L2
L3
L4
S2
S1
L5
KIDNEY ZONES
POSTERIOR ASPECT
LEFT KIDNEY
C.2
C3
C4
T.2
T.3
T.4
T.5
T.6
T.7
T.8
T.9
T.10
T.11
T.12
C.5
T.1
L.1
L.2
S.3
L.3
S.2
S.1
L4
S.1

FIG. 61

Zones affected

The segments involved are usually only on the affected side from T.8 to T.12 and L.1 to L.3 with a maximal point in T.4, radiating into C.3 to C.4.

IN THE BACK. Tension is particularly increased lateral to the vertebral column in the segments T.8 to T.12 and L.1 to L.3. A very tense area can often be observed which passes from the vertebral column lateral to the latissimus dorsi border in the segments T.9 to T.10. The area between scapula and spinal column in T.4 seems to be related to lower thoracic segments which are affected. Treatment of this point often releases the lower tension areas. The cervical segments affected pass over the trapezius border.

IN FRONT. The tension over the pelvic region is continued forward over the iliac crest into the groin and along the ilio-tibial tract. An area which often gives discomfort is to be found above the patella in L.3.

Treatment

The treatment is started in sitting with the basic section, omitting on the affected side the subcostal strokes. Here an exception is made to the general rule that all treatment should progress from caudal to cranialward, and the maximal point between scapula and spine is already included in the early treatment sessions. It is, however, very important to treat this area carefully with flat strokes, avoiding depth at first. A return to the basic section often shows improvement in the tension over the subcostal region. The strokes are carried from the medial border of the scapula diagonally up towards the vertebral column. The buttock region is treated in side lying, while the areas of the ilio-tibial tract are best treated in lying. Strokes over rectus femoris and the vasti, converging on to the patella, will soon give relief over this area. The treatment is terminated by carrying the strokes over the iliac crest down towards the symphysis pubis. It will in most cases be advisable to concentrate in the first two or three treatments on the basic section and the buttock regions in order to relieve tension in these areas.

BLADDER

Connective tissue massage may prove beneficial for patients who have passed through an acute inflammatory condition of the bladder or who suffer from a chronic catarrhal condition of the bladder. Both types of patients are inclined to suffer from discomfort or even pain when the feet get cold or wet. These patients often suffer permanently from cold feet and find it very difficult to get them warm in the evening in bed. The feeling of cold is often typically described as going up as far as the knee. Patients complain of superficial sensitivity of the sacral area, the buttock region, especially over the ischial tuberosity, along the ilio-tibial tract, in the peripheral distribution of the lumbar segments in front of the thigh and in the popliteal space. Morning stiffness which takes some time to wear off is also often a distressing symptom. The segments affected are always the lumbar and sacral segments 1 to 3 and often the increased tissue tension reaches into the lower thoracic segments.

IN THE BACK. Tension is particularly increased over the lower part of the sacrum in the segments S.2 to S.3, along the ilio-tibial tract and in the peripheral distribution of the segments L.3 and S.1 to S.2 over the popliteal fossa.

IN FRONT. Tension is specially increased over the pubic superior rami in the segment L.1 and L.2, areas in front of the thigh in the segments L.2 to L.3 and a little lower in segments L.3 to L.4.

Treatment

The treatment is started with the basic section in sitting and it will rarely be necessary to progress into higher segments. Concentration on the sacral area is essential and the buttock region is best treated in the side-lying position. The thigh region must be treated in lying. It is sometimes difficult to obtain the cutting reaction over the ilio-tibial tract, and a return to the region of the iliac crest and stimulation of the area of the trigonum lumborum is necessary. Treatment of the posterior aspect of the great trochanter region and the area between ischial tuberosity and anal cleft will eventually result in a

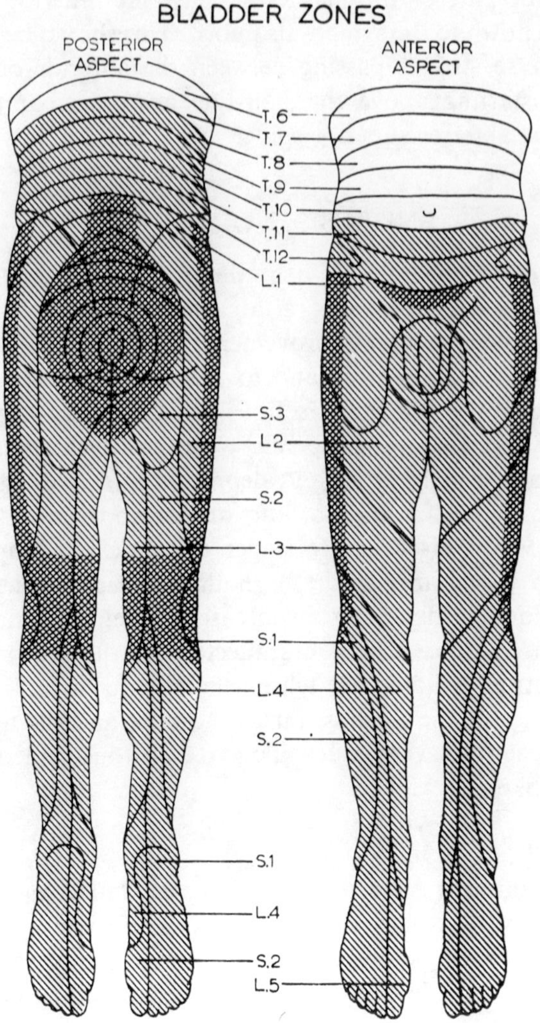

FIG. 62

satisfactory reaction. Treatment of the latter area often results in sudden pain phenomena comparable to lumbago which can easily be removed by strokes in the lumbar area. In order to normalize the tissue tension anteriorly and posteriorly the treatment should be terminated by carrying the strokes over the anterior part of the iliac crest, past the anterior superior iliac spine down to the symphysis pubis. This should be followed by transverse strokes passing between the anterior borders of the iliae, starting above the hair-line and terminating at the level of the anterior superior spines.

ENURESIS NOCTURNA

It is often possible to help these children, unless severe organic pathology is present, although in such cases it is sometimes possible to obtain improvement. It is essential to educate the mother simultaneously and to prevent punishment in case of accidents. In cases of serious psychological disturbance, it will be necessary to co-operate with the psychiatrist. These children are usually timid and depressed and it is essential to gain their confidence and not hurt or disturb them. It is therefore important in the early stages to work very superficially but touch very firmly at the beginning of each stroke because these children suffer from an intense tickling sensation at the slightest irritation. The zones affected are the typical bladder zones, but the children are tense generally and unable to relax. The muscles of the thigh as far as the knee and the muscles of the abdomen are very much increased in tone and often give a cramp-like appearance.

Treatment

The treatment is started with the basic section and is carried out in forward lying, which must be made very comfortable by support with pillows under the groin. Only short lifting strokes of very little depth should be used, avoiding in the early two to three treatments any long strokes, which may be very painful or result in a severe tickling sensation. This applies particularly to the iliac crest and the subcostal area. The latter is best avoided in the early treatments. It is important to treat the whole buttock area and particularly the areas of the great trochanter of the femur and the ilio-tibial tract. The treatment of the tract must be continued into the popliteal fossa, and stretching of this area will usually prove helpful. Gradually the treatment should be progressed into the thoracic region with particular attention to the maximal point of the kidney in T.4. It should be possible to reach this area in approximately three to four treatments and proceed into the lower abdominal region by treating, in lying, the pubic area at the termination of each treatment session. The strokes applied should cover the anterior part of the iliac crest, continuing down to the symphysis pubis and the area between the anterior borders of the iliae by transverse strokes up to the level of the anterior superior iliac spines. These latter strokes must be applied initially with fingers at a very acute angle in order to avoid depth. The treatment time with children should not exceed twenty to thirty minutes. To start with at least three sessions per week are advisable, gradually decreasing the treatment frequency. When the children start to have undisturbed nights it will still be advisable to continue the treatment until approximately twelve to fifteen sessions have been carried out.

GYNAECOLOGICAL AND OBSTETRIC CONDITIONS

Most of the pathological conditions of the organs of reproduction, particularly in the female, cause either reflex disturbances in the function of these organs or pain symptoms in the peripheral distribution of the sacral and lumbar nerves. Backache is one of the outstanding symptoms in many of these patients. Previous investigation will have eliminated a number of patients in whom the backache is either of orthopaedic origin or is caused by pathological changes in one or the other of the pelvic organs, such as the uterus, ovaries, etc. There remain, however, a number of female patients in whom no pathological condition of the organ can be found, while the functional disturbance (*e.g.* dysmenorrhoea) or the pain in the lower back and limbs resists various forms of treatment. Another group of patients suffers from persistent backache after gynaecological operations which removed the organic pathology. The backache cannot be improved by the usual methods of treatment by various forms of heat and exercises. It is for these conditions that C.T.M. is the treatment of choice, and in many cases gives excellent results. It is important to stress that any treatment which concentrates on the sacral area and is aiming for a reflex effect will stimulate the pelvic outflow of the autonomic nervous system. It is therefore essential that the physiotherapist works in very close co-operation with the doctor in charge of the patient and gives frequent reports about the patient's progress and reaction.

The conditions which in many cases derive great benefit from C.T.M. can be grouped under menstrual disturbances, post-operative symptoms after gynaecological pathology, various disturbances of pregnancy, labour and puerperium, and persistent peripheral pain after the resolution of pelvic inflammatory processes. A variety of symptomatic disturbances of the climacterium also respond very well to C.T.M.

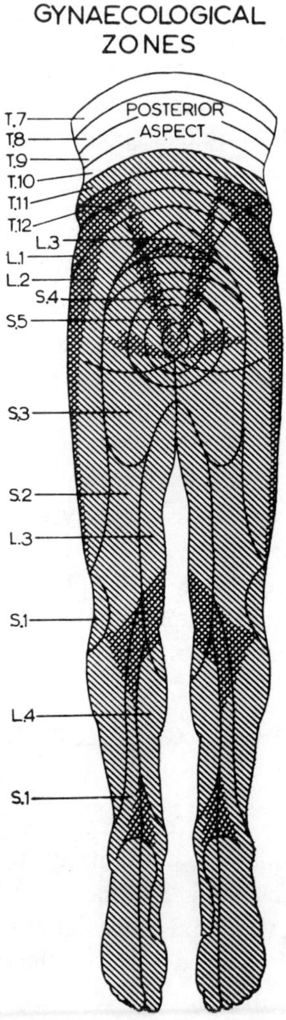

FIG. 63

The zones affected are to be found in the segments T.11 to T.12, L.1 to L.5 and S.1 to S.5. Additional connective tissue zones in other parts of the body may be found in conditions due to climacteric disturbances of the endocrine system.

MENSTRUAL DISTURBANCES

Amenorrhoea

The absence of the menstrual period may often be due to psychological upsets in young women and could be observed particularly during the war and before the war in continental countries under Nazi occupation. The sacral area appears remarkably flat as the tissue over the sacrum is increased in tension. The borders of the sacrum and the areas over the dorsum ilii appear drawn in.

Treatment

The treatment is started in the sitting position by stimulating the trigger points of this area, *i.e.* (1) the trigonum lumborum, (2) the posterior border of the great trochanter of the femur, (3) the area medial to the ischial tuberosity. Each stimulating stroke is repeated three or four times. (The patient must be warned of the very sharp shock-like pain which may result.) This is followed by the basic section with emphasis on the angle between sacrum and iliae. Should no cutting reaction be obtained, a return to the trigger points will give the desired result. This is followed by treatment of the anterior pelvic area in lying. Strokes are applied from the anterior part of the iliac crest towards the symphysis pubis, followed by transverse strokes between the anterior borders of the iliae. As soon as tension permits the posterior aspect of the sacrum is treated during the basic section by transverse strokes passing between the posterior sacral foraminae. The treatment should be repeated on four to five consecutive days, followed by a rest period of ten days. Should menstruation occur during this period, the whole sequence is repeated two weeks before the next period is due; otherwise it is repeated after the ten days' interval. According to the German authors, beneficial results are to be expected in most cases of functional amenorrhoea. The treatment should be repeated for three to four months in order to normalize function again. As previously mentioned, no treatment is ever given during a menstrual period.

Dysmenorrhoea

The patients usually complain of severe backache in the sacral region, very often accompanied by constipation. Tension areas can be observed over the sacrum and the dorsum iliae. In some cases a liver zone can also be seen.

Treatment

The treatment is carried out as previously described for amenorrhoea except that trigger points should not be stimulated. It is advisable to include in the treatment the latissimus dorsi border and the intercostal spaces up to T.7. Treatment should be started two weeks before the date of the next menstrual period, two to three times during the first week and daily during the second week. As soon as the menstrual discharge ceases treatment should be resumed, at first once or twice a week, and then the previously described cycle is repeated. Painless menstrual periods can be expected confidently after approximately fifteen treatments, when the tension in the connective tissue zones should have considerably improved unless a definite pathological condition is present. Before terminating the C.T.M. treatment, the patient should be taught localized pelvic tilting (Kohlrausch and Leube, 1933) exercises, to be practised regularly during the two weeks preceding the menstrual period.

Climacteric Disturbances

These may produce a variety of symptoms such as low backache, particularly present during the later part of the night and on getting up, digestive disturbances, headaches, paraesthesia of arms and legs and facial flushes. Many of these patients appear generally depressed, listless and tired. Connective tissue massage applied particularly to the basic and thoracic sections with emphasis on the subcostal region very often produces dramatic results. One of the consultants for whom the author worked used to speak of "euphoria" replacing the previous rather gloomy outlook on life.

Pregnancy

The German authors (Dicke, 1953) claim that " infantile uterus " can be improved by the application of C.T.M. to such an extent that conception and pregnancy occur, sometimes after years of disappointment. The author has personally known of a case where a variety of medical treatments were unsuccessful. The application of C.T.M. to the sacral and lumbar regions resulted very soon in a pregnancy which unfortunately was terminated by a miscarriage. Several years passed without conception until C.T.M. was again applied. This time a pregnancy occurred with a normal delivery of a healthy infant.

Some of the symptomatic discomforts of pregnancy, such as circulatory disturbances, particularly in the legs, and sciatic pain can be treated with C.T.M. without any danger (Teirich-Leube, 1960). The areas to be treated are the lateral borders of the sacrum, the posterior aspect of the great trochanter of the femur (in side lying) and the ilio-tibial tract (in lying). Antenatal exercises (Ebner, 1982) carefully taught for home practice will also help to overcome the circulatory difficulties.

Labour

German authors (Dicke, 1953; Teirich-Leube, 1960) mention the beneficial results which can be obtained by the application of C.T.M.

Some difficulties that may arise are: a) Insufficient strength of contractions b) Lack of relaxation and slow progress in the taking up of the lower uterine segment.

The strokes are applied to the lateral border and the dorsal surface of the sacrum and over the zones which usually show tension changes in menstrual disturbances over the lower lumbar region. (Ebner–Risk, 1972). From German colleagues the author has received information that delayed delivery is sometimes speeded up by doctors using the technique. It is used in Germany by doctors for diagnostic as well as therapeutic purposes.

Lactation

One of the factors contributing to successful breast-feeding is an adequate capillary blood supply to the mammary gland. Another is the mother's ability to manage successfully and serenely the demands of her daily life. Feeding difficulties, therefore, often arise when the mother returns home. Under these circumstances C.T.M. proves very beneficial. The areas to be treated in sitting are the basic and thoracic sections, including latissimus dorsi and the axilla. In lying the pelvic and costal strokes are continued forward as far as the rectus abdominis. One or two additional simple exercises in the form of shoulder rolling with emphasis on complete flexion in the shoulder joint (pectoralis major action) will enhance the value of the C.T.M.

Hysterectomy and other Gynaecological Operations

Patients who have undergone these operations are often troubled by backache and/or circulatory disturbances in the legs and feet. The legs feel heavy and the areas round the ankles are swollen. All these patients improve considerably with C.T.M. which helps to re-establish the autonomic balance. For these patients the treatment should be carried out in forward lying for the back regions and in lying for the treatment of the thighs. It is usually unnecessary to include the lower legs in the treatment. Re-education of correct postural habits must be attempted simultaneously as the back pain will otherwise return.

CHAPTER XII

Neurological Conditions

IT is important to realize that in most neurological conditions return to full health is impossible. Pathological changes have taken place and must be accepted as irreversible. Modern physiology has, however, made it clear that all systems of the human body normally work only to a fraction of their capacity and possess enormous stores of reserve power. The treatment by physiotherapeutic agents of neurological conditions must therefore aim at functional rehabilitation. All tissues of the human body depend for their function on an adequate blood supply and it is in this way that C.T.M. may represent a very valuable adjunct to exercise therapy. Both main groups of neurological conditions, *i.e.* upper motor neuron lesions and lower motor neuron lesions, show severe symptoms of interference with the blood supply of the affected parts. Recent research has shown that the highest centres of autonomic control may be found in the cerebral cortex and the mid-brain, which explains the marked circulatory changes in the affected limbs in conditions such as hemiplegia. In lower motor neuron lesions the interference with the circulation occurs at spinal level. The axons of the lateral horn cells pass through the anterior horn and emerge from the spinal cord via the anterior root. All inflammatory or degenerative processes which take place in the lower motor centres will therefore affect to a certain extent the autonomic spinal fibres. This explains the circulatory changes which take place in the affected parts in conditions such as anterior poliomyelitis. Afferent pathways not only play a very important part in the performance of voluntary movement but are equally important in circulatory reactions. It is also important to consider the fact that all tissues with diminished blood supply show a tendency to degenerate into fibrous tissue which in time is inclined to become more avascular and contract. This may partly explain the tendency to contracture which so often is a complicating symptom in all types of nerve lesion. Another symptom in all cases of diminished peripheral blood supply is the lack of adaptation to external thermal stimuli producing complications in the form of chilblains and ulcers. Connective tissue massage can help considerably to stimulate peripheral pathways. In the author's experience it is possible to avoid frost damage during the winter months in patients suffering from infantile paralysis. In other conditions, such as disseminated sclerosis, and Parkinsons Disease the massage promotes relaxation and improves muscle function. A small selection of typical nerve lesions will be discussed below in order to describe the rationale of the application of C.T.M. The adaptation to other lesions should not, therefore, present any difficulty.

This introduction would not be complete without drawing the Reader's attention to the outstanding contribution which had been made by the work of Bobath (Reference: Bobath). It has opened a new field of rehabilitation for neurological pathology.

ANTERIOR POLIOMYELITIS

Treatment

The treatment should be started when the general hyperaesthesia is subsiding, *i.e.* approximately three weeks after the acute onset. It is important to start the treatment as soon as possible in order to minimize peripheral circulatory disturbances. It must be remembered that these not only influence muscle action but also affect the growth of structures such as bone in children. The treatment is given in the recumbent position and starts with the basic section. Progression into upper segments is only carried out if the upper limbs or the back or abdominal muscles are affected. Early treatment sessions should not exceed fifteen minutes in order to avoid fatigue. It is important to follow the massage with at least two full-range movements of all joints in the body, as increased connective tissue tension in one part of the body may cause tension changes in other parts. As recovery progresses the length of treatment time can be increased. The affected autonomic fibres come from the spinal cord and it is therefore important to make use of all peripheral reflexes and of reflex centres which lie outside the cord. As soon as pain sensibility permits, the affected limbs should, therefore, be included in the treatment. It is important in the lower limb to stress special connective tissue structures such as the gluteal fascia, the ilio-tibial tract, popliteal fascia, all structures connected to the tendo achillis and the plantar fascia; in the upper limb all structures round the shoulder girdle, including the deltoid fascia, and in the hand the palmar fascia and the interosseous spaces. Special attention to full finger extension is important. If the intercostal muscles are affected careful attention must be paid to the treatment of the full length of each intercostal space. Treatment of this area should be followed immediately with localized breathing exercises. It is necessary to graduate the depth of strokes very carefully so as not to cause pain to the patient. It has proved very beneficial to add C.T.M. to the treatment programme of patients who have suffered the acute attack several years ago and are particularly troubled in the cold season by circulatory disturbances.

CASE 16. Female, aged 5. *Diagnosis :* Anterior poliomyelitis. From the patient's case papers the following history was obtained. In May 1952 the child became ill, vomited and showed signs of paralysis of the right leg. At this stage she was admitted to a hospital for infectious diseases. After three weeks the child was discharged to an orthopaedic hospital where it was found that the anterior abdominal muscles were quite strong so that she could lift her head easily; the lateral group of abdominal muscles, however, showed some weakness. The right leg showed severe paralysis. The hip flexors were very weak; only tensor fascia femoris could act against gravity. The quadriceps muscles and hamstrings showed only a flicker of movement. The rest of the lower limb was quite flail. At this stage the limb was immobilized in plaster of Paris. Two months later the abdominal muscles had improved so that they could act against gravity; the rest of the affected muscles showed no improvement. At this stage the patient started exercises in the pool and could progress to walking with a caliper three weeks later. After a period of a further four weeks the child left the hospital in order to attend for further physiotherapy treatment as an out-patient. She could now walk with a caliper and was wearing a Glassonia corset. A year later the corset could be discarded. When the orthopaedic consultant prescribed C.T.M. in December 1959, the child had suffered every winter since 1952 from chilblains in the lower half of the right calf and on the toes. The leg felt cold and dead even in the summer. Protective covering with cotton-wool in the winter months could not prevent ulceration of the chilblains. On investigation it was found that the back and the left buttock appeared normal, the right leg appeared cold and the lower half of the right calf was blue with old chilblain marks. The right buttock arterial zone + + +.

Treatment

1. Basic section treated. Reflex sensation and erythema were easily obtained. Half an hour after termination of the treatment the leg had a warm glow.
2. The leg was cold on arrival but the patient reported that the warm glow had lasted for twenty-four hours. Basic section treated. The leg was warm again after treatment.
3. The patient reported that the warmth in the leg had lasted for twenty-four hours, while the thigh felt warm for two days. Basic section treated.
4. The child reported that her leg now felt "live" and light and the warmth had lasted in the whole limb for two days. On arrival the leg was cold but less blue. Basic section treated.
5. The patient reported that the whole limb including the foot had felt warm and remained so for three days. Basic section treated.
6. On arrival the leg and foot were warm. Basic section treated.
7. On arrival the limb was warm and the child reported that the leg tired less easily. Same areas treated.
8. On arrival the limb felt warm to the patient and was warm to the touch as far as the middle of the calf. Basic section and the thigh as far as the popliteal space treated. After termination of the treatment the whole limb, including the toes, was warm to touch and the colour of the calf had changed to dark pink.
9. The limb was warm on arrival. Same areas treated.

Six further treatments were given to the same areas. The limb always felt warm and the colour was steadily improving. The chilblain marks became fainter.

16. Three further treatments were given to the same areas at weekly intervals.
19. The appearance of the leg was now normal and the chilblain marks had disappeared. Same areas treated. The treatment interval was now increased to two weeks. Same areas treated.

On termination of the course of treatments (twenty-four) the patient's leg now always felt warm, comfortable and light. She was reviewed by the orthopaedic consultant six weeks later and it was found that her leg was quite warm and showed no discolouration. The patient reported that it had been exposed to cold winds without being discoloured.

SCIATICA

Pain in the origin and distribution of the sciatic nerve may be due to a variety of causes, and careful diagnosis will have eliminated a number of patients unsuitable for treatment by C.T.M. This refers particularly to patients in whom the source of the pain is pressure inside the pelvis or direct pressure on the nerve roots. Conditions of this kind include pelvic tumours, acute gynaecological inflammatory conditions, inflammatory condition of the spinal column, and inflammatory conditions of the cord, such as tabes, etc. There remain, however, a number of patients suffering from sciatic pain who will benefit greatly from the application of C.T.M. either as the sole treatment or as an adjunct to other medical or orthopaedic measures. The sciatic pain may be caused by neuritis or neuralgia of the sciatic nerve or the sacral plexus as part of a rheumatic syndrome, or it may appear as part of a toxic condition due to a focus somewhere else in the body. The pain may remain as a symptom, although the original cause has been removed due to the alteration in connective tissue tension in the areas of origin or course of the nerve. This applies particularly to gynaecological conditions which have cleared up in the course of medical or surgical intervention. Localized pelvic tilting exercises are often a valuable help in the later stages of treatment.

The sciatic nerve is formed from the lumbar-sacral trunk and includes rami from the fourth and fifth lumbar roots and from the first, second and third sacral roots. The peripheral distribution includes the greater part of the lower limb. Pain distribution is very typical. If the right sciatic nerve is affected, alterations in tissue tension can be found over the right sacro-iliac joint, in a strip of tissue running parallel to the gluteal fold and including the area of the ischial tuberosity, and in a strip of tissue between the ischial tuberosity and the great trochanter of the femur. Additionally the tissue on the left side of the spinal column at the level of the third and fourth lumbar vertebrae shows alterations in tension. According to Leube and Dicke (1948) a very frequent relationship seems to exist between this area and the area between the femoral trochanter and ischial tuberosity. Treatment of the lumbar area on the left causes paraesthetic symptoms in the right peripheral distribution in the form of " pins and needles " or numbness in the buttocks or stabbing pain round the ankle or sole of the foot. Strokes over the trochanter area almost immediately remove these symptoms. After normalization of the tension changes the symptoms caused by the apparent interrelation of these two points can no longer be elicited. Tension and pain symptoms may also be present over the upper part of the ilio-tibial tract, in the popliteal space and at the back of the calf in the upper prolongation of the tendo achillis between the two heads of gastrocnemius.

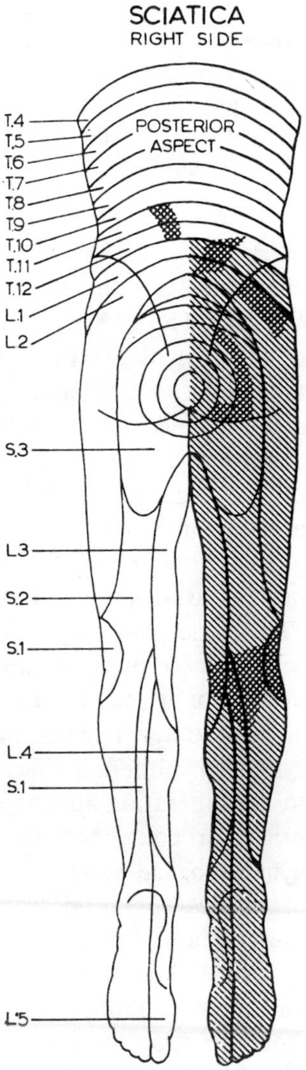

FIG. 64

Treatment

The position for treatment

must be adapted to the patient's comfort. It is advisable to treat the basic section in the sitting position, if this is possible, while the gluteal region and the lower limb are best treated in the side-lying position. The strokes must be carried out very slowly in order to obtain a cutting reaction and not cause unnecessary discomfort to the patient. It may be necessary to treat the peripheral segmental distribution but this should not be attempted in the first few treatments. Special attention should be given to the treatment of the sacro-lumbar angle, gradually increasing the length of the strokes by starting in mid-axillary line over the iliac crest. The buttock area should next be treated, at first with short lifting strokes, until it is possible to carry long strokes parallel to the iliac crest, starting at the sacro-iliac joint, passing laterally above and below the great trochanter of the femur and ending round the anterior superior iliac spine. The massage proceeds to the area between ischial tuberosity and great trochanter by strokes passing at right angles towards the posterior border of the trochanter and the ilio-tibial tract. To finish the treatment of this area long strokes are taken along the upper one-third of the ilio-tibial tract, passing upwards and round the great trochanter to finish in front. Treatment of the sacral and buttock areas very often results in the patient's report of a wave of warmth passing down the leg. Further progression of treatment should be directed towards the popliteal area by carrying strokes from the middle of the thigh laterally behind the ilio-tibial tract and medially behind the semitendinosus towards the knee and slightly forward to end just below the joint line. The two heads of gastrocnemius are stroked bimanually along their medial borders towards the popliteal space. Should discomfort be present along the lateral aspect of the lower leg, the treatment of the peroneal septum should be added. The treatment is completed in lying by strokes over the iliac crest and the posterior border of the ilio-tibial tract. No course of treatment should be terminated until the tension in the areas of the root segments is normalized and all peripheral symptoms have disappeared. It will probably be necessary to carry out twenty to thirty treatments, gradually increasing the interval between treatments. It might be advisable to carry out a short course of treatment after an interval of approximately six months in order to make certain that no tension areas have returned.

HEMIPLEGIA

It is well to remember that many patients who suffer a cerebral catastrophe may have been leading a very active life which is suddenly interrupted. As a rule, the sudden cessation of activity has not only a detrimental effect on the patient's general health, but usually also a depressing effect on the patient's morale. As soon as the patient recovers consciousness and the doctor gives permission, very short and carefully given C.T.M. may prove a very valuable adjunct to exercise therapy. It must be remembered that not only cerebral motor and sensory fibres may be involved due to the haemorrhage, but that certainly some autonomic fibres will be affected. The blue, cold limb, so distressing to the patient, is certainly not only the result of lack of movement. At first it is very difficult to predict how much recovery will take place, but it is safe to reassure the patient that some recovery will occur and that intercommunicating fibres exist so that the left side of the cerebral hemisphere can develop a certain amount of control over the left side of the body. It is therefore very important that the affected muscle groups should receive the best possible blood supply and that no contractures are allowed to develop. Connective tissue massage leaves the patient with a feeling of well-being and therefore helps to improve the general attitude of the patient towards personal co-operation which is the essential factor in the recovery process attempted by physiotherapy.

Many of these patients have suffered for a considerable time of High Blood Pressure which may have affected Kidney function. The author has treated a patient with very high Blood urea content which very quickly responded to C.T.M. As no harm can be done to the patient, it is well worth-while in these desperate cases.

Treatment

The patient is first treated in the side-lying position. Only very short treatment of the basic section (approximately ten minutes) is given first, gradually progressing into the lower limb. If the patient progresses favourably, the latissimus dorsi border is treated and progressed into the treatment of the upper limb as soon as possible. Special care must be taken to treat the shoulder area and the hand in order to avoid contractures. In order to avoid interference with the gradual recovery of the general circulation, the thoracic and cervical sections should not be treated. Exercise Therapy see Ref. Bobath.

DISSEMINATED SCLEROSIS

(Multiple Sclerosis)

The pathological process in this disease is focal demyelination, disseminated irregularly throughout the cerebrospinal axis. The disease takes its characteristic course in periods of remissions and exacerbations, and considerable functional recovery may occur during remission periods. Symptoms are very diverse due to the irregular distribution of the lesions. Some of the most constant symptoms are weakness in the dorsiflexors of one foot and fatigue after short periods of exertion. Although no remedy is known at the present time, it is impossible to forecast the future of any individual patient. A great deal of functional recovery can take place if adequate treatment is established in time. It is essential to gain the patient's confidence and co-operation, as short frequent periods of well-selected exercises are more valuable than longer treatment periods three or four times a week. These should be reserved for treatment which will improve the general health of the patient, relieve symptoms of pain which are often present in the back, and check the patient's home exercise programme. Connective tissue massage increases the patient's feeling of well-being, improves the circulation to the muscles, especially in the back, and so relieves fatigue pain. The improved circulation to the digestive organs and the liver will improve their function and contribute to general health and regular elimination of waste products.

Treatment

The basic section should be treated in sitting if back pain is not a predominant symptom, otherwise the whole treatment should be carried out in the recumbent position. During the first treatment the leg areas can be included if it is possible to obtain a cutting reaction. The depth of the strokes must be adapted to the patient's pain symptoms which under no account should be increased. The patient must be left with a feeling of comfortable warmth and relaxation. It is also important not to elicit any muscle spasm following the strokes. The increased blood supply to the limbs should produce decreased spasticity in the affected limb muscles, such as the adductors. Following the massage treatment a very short exercise session should be added, mainly for the purpose of teaching two or three home exercises and practising correct walking. It will be found that noticeable functional improvement occurs after the C.T.M. which gives encouragement to the patient. Some of the improvement (*e.g.* adductor spasm) is gradually retained so that an over-all improved function can be achieved unless a new attack occurs. The use of the Exercycle for short but frequent periods at home gives excellent results.

As soon as possible the C.T.M. should include the whole back which should remain the main area of treatment. Progression to include the upper limb is made after two or three treatments if the limb is affected. Circulatory changes in the hands, in the form of paraesthesia and blueness, can be relieved considerably. Great attention must be paid to the hands in order to avoid contractures occurring in any form. For home exercises, tennis balls or pieces of sponge rubber provide an excellent means of retaining gripping power. If a stick is used for walking it is important to draw the patient's attention to balanced muscle action in the trunk and not permit swaying of the body weight completely to one side.

CASE 17. Male, aged 48. *Occupation:* Managing Director.

Diagnosis : Multiple sclerosis. The patient started C.T.M. in October 1960 and the following history was obtained from his case papers. He had started with severe diplopia and had suffered from increasing disabilities for the past ten years. In addition to increasing walking difficulties due to muscle spasm and inco-ordination, he suffered from severe trigeminal neuralgia. All teeth were extracted and the lowest branch of the nerve injected with alcohol. In the autumn of 1959 he had had a course of injections with very severe reaction, consisting of very high fever and inability to pass water voluntarily. The bladder difficulty had resolved itself after several weeks.

On investigation it was found that both feet were cold and blue, the right more so than the left. The right leg showed over-all extensor and adductor spasm, and voluntary hip-knee flexion was impossible but could be obtained as a mass movement by passively bending the big toe into plantar flexion. Over the ankle joint only extensor hallucis worked voluntarily. In the left leg voluntary but weak hip-knee flexion was possible and the ankle joint possessed sufficient voluntary dorsiflexion to clear the ground easily. In both upper limbs the shoulder and elbow movements were functionally normal. The left hand showed no disability but was frequently cold and blue. The right hand was always blue and cold, the little finger and ring finger felt numb to the patient, and the muscles of the ulnar supply were affected, giving the appearance of a *main en griffe*. Voluntary gripping power was quite good and the patient could write. The abdominal muscles, especially on the right side, were weak and the patient could only get out of bed or change from sitting to standing with the help of the arm flexors. His speech was slurred.

Treatment

1. Basic section, latissimus dorsi and all four limbs treated. A good circulatory response was obtained with slight wheal formation in the back. The strokes in the lower extremity were very sharp. After the massage weak voluntary hip-knee flexion with the right leg was possible, the right hand felt warm and the numbness in the ulnar two fingers was slightly improved. At this stage the patient was advised to buy an Exercycle for daily practice in the morning and evening. A Rizzoli splint was ordered for the right leg to prevent foot-drop during walking.
2. The patient reported that he went to sleep one and a half hours after the last treatment while watching television. Same areas treated, with the additional inclusion of the

back to the level of T.7. After the massage free hip-knee flexion in the lying position in both limbs was possible. In sitting the left thigh could be raised from the chair and change from sitting to standing was possible without assistance. The patient was advised to practise these exercises several times for short periods during the day.

3. The previously attained functional movements were still possible. Same areas treated, with additional inclusion of the back to the level of C.7. The back felt warm and comfortable after the treatment and the adductor spasm in the right leg had decreased. Re-education of correct walking was started.
4. Same areas treated.
5. The patient was found to be very depressed because of frequent attacks of trigeminal neuralgic pain. Same areas and the whole back to the occiput treated. No attack of neuralgia occurred during the treatment. The patient was left relaxed and freely talking.
6. The attacks of trigeminal neuralgia had been less frequent and less severe during the treatment interval (three days). Same areas treated and the exercise programme carried out by the patient as described.

Two further treatments were given on the same lines.

9. The patient reported that after the massage he could now dress himself without assistance; friends remarked that he was looking much better and his speech was no longer slurred. Same areas treated.

Three further treatments were carried out on the same lines.

13. The patient reported that he had had no attacks of trigeminal neuralgia for over a week. His back felt more mobile but slightly painful after a full day's work. He mentioned that he drove the car for a short distance and could handle the brake with the right hand. Same areas treated. The exercise programme was increased by adding static contractions to the postural muscles in the back. The Exercycle had been obtained and the patient had been advised to practise for one minute two to three times per day. During the following three weeks the treatment was continued on the same lines twice a week. After the massage the functional movements could be carried out much more easily and some of the improvement was retained during the treatment intervals.
20. The patient reported that he had had a slight attack of influenza and was distressed by constipation. Same areas

treated, with emphasis on the liver area.

21. The patient reported that his bowels opened half an hour after termination of the massage. He complained of diffuse pain in the back and the right arm with numbness in all finger-tips of the right hand. Same areas treated. After the treatment sensation had returned to all finger-tips except that of the little finger.

The treatment was continued on the same lines twice weekly during the following seven weeks when the patient went on holiday. At that stage the slow functional improvement of movement had been maintained in spite of cold weather. The backache had been controlled by paying attention to postural contractions and a change of chair in the factory. The speech was no longer slurred unless the patient was very tired.

The future programme for this patient will continue on the lines described in this case history. His general health is greatly improved during the periods when he is receiving C.T.M. The marked increase in functional ability after the treatment has a very beneficial influence on his general morale. It makes it possible for him to continue with his occupation and remain independent. A very important aspect is that the patient knows from experience that the treatment will help him during difficult periods.

PARALYSIS AGITANS

(Parkinson's Disease)

Nothing definite is known of the factors which lead to the development of this disease. It is probable that it represents a local senile degeneration in the cells and fibre tracts of some of the basal ganglia. A clinical picture closely resembling the symptoms of paralysis agitans often follows the inflammatory lesions of epidemic encephalitis. The true disease usually occurs in middle-aged or old people, while the encephalitic variety may be present in the younger age groups. There are two main clinical types: one in whom muscular rigidity is the prominent symptom, while tremor is inconstant and not very troublesome; the other in whom tremor is the most disabling symptom throughout the course of the disease. As the extrapyramidal fibres to the anterior horn cells are pathologically affected the outstanding symptoms are connected with interference of impulses conveying co-ordination, balance, emotional attitudes, facial expressions and postural tone. From the patient's point of view there is an increasing loss of automatic movement, decrease of muscle power, difficulty in carrying out the movements of daily living (*e.g.* getting up from a chair), difficulty in facial expression (mask-like face) and often aching pains, particularly in the shoulders and arms. The back and chest feel encased in a rigid jacket and this state interferes with respiration and consequently the general health of the patient. The absence of the incessant adaptive movements of daily life and the increasing difficulty of carrying out voluntary exercise seriously interfere with the circulation which partly depends on the pumping action of muscles. The decrease of reflex and voluntary activity therefore aggravates the circulatory situation. New Drug-therapy and modern surgical treatment seem to hold out new hope for some of these patients. In all cases movement re-education, relaxation and breathing exercises are essential. The effect of these therapeutic measures can be greatly enhanced by giving C.T.M. prior to these forms of therapy. It is very rewarding to hear from these patients the expression of relief when the tightness round the thorax is released and breathing becomes easier. A patient used the expression: "It feels like having armour removed from your chest." Both sleep and digestion improve and therefore the patient's mental attitude becomes more hopeful.

Treatment

The treatment is concentrated on the back. Basic, cervical and thoracic sections should be treated as soon as possible. During the treatment of the thoracic section in the back, the anterior aspect of the thorax should also be included in the treatment. After approximately four to six treatments progression can be made to include the limbs. The mask-like face responds very well to facial strokes as described in the chapters on technique.

It is very important to counteract the tendency to flexion contractures which exists in these patients not only by exercises but also by stretching manipulations as previously described in the axilla, the elbow and the popliteal fossa. When the whole body has been included in the C.T.M. treatment, it is advisable to arrange it in sections in order to avoid fatigue. One session should treat the basic section and the lower limbs. the next session should only quickly pass through the basic section area and concentrate on the thoracic and cervical sections including the upper limbs. A rest period after the treatment proves very beneficial and is often followed by restful sleep. Weighted pendular swinging exercises for home practise should be taught.

SUBACUTE COMBINED DEGENERATION OF THE CORD

This is a disease associated with pernicious anaemia in which progressive degeneration of the posterior and lateral columns of the spinal cord occurs. The peripheral nerves also undergo degenerative changes. The nervous symptoms may precede the clinical manifestation of the blood disease. If this is not the case the nervous symptoms appear in the early stages of the pernicious anaemia. The degenerative changes first affect the myelin sheaths and later follow degeneration of the axis cylinder. Clinically two main types of nerve symptoms may be observed, although transitional stages between the two extreme types may be found. The one type reveals primarily weakness in the peripheral distribution of motor nerves with impairment of cutaneous sensibility, especially to touch. There is always, however, a certain amount of involvement of the posterior columns which explains the symptoms of postural instability and a certain amount of ataxic gait. Later the pyramidal tracts also become involved and give symptoms of an upper motor neuron lesion. This type with primary involvement of peripheral nerves shows much better prospects of recovery. The second type gives at first the picture of a spastic paresis with most symptoms of an upper motor neuron lesion. Peripheral muscular weakness and sensory symptoms follow later. The prospect of recovery is far less hopeful. Respiratory symptoms, such as breathlessness, are often associated with the blood condition. Clinically the patient presents a picture of yellowish pallor. She complains of fatigue after very little exertion, the legs feel heavy and weak, and the hands are clumsy and unable to carry out fine movements. The patient also reports various forms of paraesthesia, such as numbness, "pins and needles" and a feeling of cotton-wool in the feet when walking barefoot.

The primary treatment is, of course, the treatment of the blood condition. As soon as the red-cell count and the haemoglobin index approach normal levels and can be maintained, the nervous condition will start to improve. Physiotherapeutic measures can help considerably to hasten the recovery and make it functionally more satisfactory for the patient. Carefully selected exercises for the affected muscle groups should be taught for home practice. This is very important as the patient can only practise for short periods until the exercise tolerance is gradually increased. Connective tissue massage helps to improve the peripheral circulation and the general health of the patient by stimulating the circulation to the respiratory and digestive organs.

Treatment

In the early stages the treatment can be carried out in lying if the patient tires easily. It starts with the basic section and is progressed as soon as possible over the whole back. The inclusion of the limbs in the treatment depends on the severity of the symptoms and the speed of recovery. If respiratory symptoms are present the anterior aspect of the chest must be included. In the early stages of treatment the patient should be treated three times per week and the frequency gradually decreased. Between thirty and fifty treatments may be necessary to give a satisfactory result.

CASE 18. Female, aged 50. *Occupation :* Housewife. Three months prior to the beginning of C.T.M. pernicious anaemia and subacute combined degeneration of the cord had been diagnosed. From the patient's case papers it had been learned that she complained of feeling dizzy when walking, that her feet and hands felt completely numb and that she was suffering from bronchitis and asthma. She had received cytamen injections once per week. On investigation it was found that very little mobility existed in the superficial tissues of the back. The patient complained of frequent attacks of severe headaches; the movements of the head were found to be very limited and painful.

Treatment

1. Basic section treated in the sitting position. All strokes were severely cutting and a good erythema was obtained.
2. Basic section treated. During the treatment the patient felt a tingling sensation in the feet and hands. After the treatment the patient volunteered the information that the back felt warm for the first time for months and that the feet felt warmer. She could feel a little sensation in the finger-tips.
3. On arrival the patient reported that the numbness in the finger-tips returned half an hour after leaving the hospital but the back continued to feel warm. Basic section treated. After the termination of the treatment the hands felt warmer and a little less numb.
4. The patient reported that the numbness in the fingers did not return until she reached home, and she felt less pain in the neck, but the rest of the back was still very painful. The treatment of the back was extended to T.7.
5. The patient reported that the back had been pain-free for the rest of the day. The following day she suffered from a very bad headache. The treatment was progressed to the occiput and both scapular areas included.
6. The patient reported that she had felt much better during the intervening three days; the headaches had been milder and less frequent. The numbness in the fingers was less severe and the hands felt warmer. Same areas treated.
7. The patient reported that she felt much better generally, the hands were cold on arrival and the feet and legs were cold as far as the knee. Same areas treated and the massage progressed to include the arms and hands.
8. The patient had felt generally comfortable during the three days' interval, but had been troubled with bronchitis. Same areas treated and the massage progressed to include the anterior aspect of the chest.
9. The patient reported that she had less pain in the back and neck, suffered less frequently from headaches, felt less dizzy, and the sensation in the fingers had begun to return. The bronchitis and coldness in the knees were still troublesome.

The next eight treatments were given to the same areas. The patient reported that the asthma had started to improve since the anterior chest region had been included in the treatment.

18. Same areas treated and the massage progressed to include the legs. After the treatment the patient reported that the legs felt warmer and that she could feel some sensation returning.
19. The patient reported that the legs felt better for a whole day following the last treatment but were very painful the next day in bed. Same areas treated.
20. The patient reported that the legs and feet felt warm for two days after the previous treatment.

The next four treatments were given to the same areas.

25. The patient reported that she was suffering very little from headaches. The right hand felt completely normal, the left hand felt slightly numb, the knees and feet were much warmer; she had increased sensation in the right foot, but still experienced a " dead " feeling in the left heel and the lateral toes of the same foot. The bronchitis and asthma were much improved.

The next three treatments were given to the same areas.

29. The legs showed a definite improvement in the circulation. The patient volunteered the statement that " she had never been as well as now." Same areas treated. During the last nineteen treatments faradism to the quadriceps had been given after the C.T.M. in order to give muscle contraction without causing fixator muscle fatigue.
30. The patient reported that she had suffered from a bad headache during the last week-end and that the legs again felt cold. Same areas treated, but faradism was discontinued.
31. The patient reported that she had been free from headache. Same areas treated.
32. The patient reported that the feet felt warm and less numb.

The next two treatments were given to the same areas.

35. The left hand, leg and foot were cold on arrival. Same areas treated. The patient reported that the limbs felt warm after the C.T.M.
36. The patient reported that the improved temperature in the left limbs lasted for one day. Same areas treated and the temperature again improved after the treatment.
37. On arrival the feet and legs were warm in spite of a cold day. Same areas treated. After the treatment the patient reported that she had a sensation of " pins and needles " in the heel of the left foot. She mentioned that sensation had been completely absent for over a year.
38. The patient reported that she felt warm " all over." Same areas treated.
39. The patient reported that during the week-end the knees

again felt cold and more "woolly." Same areas treated. After the first few sacral strokes the legs felt warm and more normal again.

Three more treatments were given to the same areas.

On termination of the course of treatment (forty-two) the general health of the patient had greatly improved, and the asthma attacks had become less frequent and less severe. Both legs felt warm and she could walk reasonable distances; the soles of the feet had still a slight feeling of cotton-wool. The right hand was completely normal; the left hand had occasional attacks of slight numbness. The patient reported that she could again knit and use her hands for all small movements. The grip in both hands was very good.

CEREBRAL PALSY

The cause of cerebral palsy in children is partly unknown and partly associated with pre-natal infectious disease of the mother or with injury to the head during birth, causing a variety of cerebral haemorrhages. Cerebral anoxia following the stretching, bending and compression of cerebral vessels may be another factor. The injury may, therefore, take place in unpredictable parts of the brain tissue and very often produces the circulatory symptoms associated with adult cerebral injury. The affected limbs are very often blue and cold when exposed to colder temperatures. Although the re-education of movement patterns and daily living functions is the most important part of the treatment of these children, the warming up of the affected parts prior to exercise therapy proves a valuable part of the treatment. Connective tissue massage proves very helpful, particularly as it demands very little preparation and can be given in most circumstances.

Treatment

The superficial tissues are very resistant to the passage of the working fingers and it is therefore advisable to work very slowly. The child is treated in the recumbent position and the massage treatment session should not exceed ten to fifteen minutes. The treatment starts with the basic section and progresses into the lower limbs if these are affected. Stretching of the popliteal space and the plantar fascia is essential in these patients. In all cases where the upper limbs are affected the treatment is progressed up the back and into the upper limb. Again special attention should be paid to the stretching of the axillary space, the antecubital fossa and the palmar fascia. It is thus possible not only to achieve better results from the exercise therapy but also to avoid chilblains which often occur in these children during the winter months. (Ref. Bobath)

CHAPTER XIII

Sports Injuries

THE treatment of sport injuries including dancing, athletics, gymnastics, games and Winter sports, has almost become a medical speciality. This is not always beneficial to the patient. The reason for this attitude is the fact that apparently the majority of these patients have suffered some trauma during physical activity, and the therapeutic effort is concentrated primarily on the injured part. It is however very important to apply the principle of the global approach also to these patients. The first consideration must be to discover how seriously the patient was involved in the activity, if it was carried out on a competitive basis, if the patient is an amateur or professional, if he belongs to a group of people who undergo regular training or if he practises the activity only to occupy his leisure periods. All these factors will influence his co-operative efforts during the recovery period. They will also influence his mental attitude, the therapeutic approach and the state of his physical capabilities prior to the injury.

There are two main groups of performers:

1) The athlete who performs within the normal optimal capability of the human body, *e.g.* the long distance runner. He has to develop during well guided training a certain amount of muscle strength and mobility in the upper and lower limbs, never beyond the optimal capacity of these structures. The main qualities to be developed are endurance of muscles and breathing control. No structure however will be used beyond its optimum.

2) The athlete or dancer who performs beyond the normal optimal capability of the human body, *e.g.* the dancer or gymnast. Normally joints are protected by ligaments which possess stretch receptors which are alerted if the joint is moved beyond its optimal range. As a result of this stimulation, certain muscles contract to prevent the excess movement. If the muscle is not strong enough to prevent the movement because of the applica-

tion of an outside force such as perpendicular swing, the muscle will tear. This factor must be known to the Therapist because the true injury may be some distance away from the affected joint. A ligmentous injury without muscle tear is impossible.

The Author had a most revealing experience during a short period when she was responsible for the therapeutic care of the members of a Ballet Company. There were daily occurrences of muscle tears. This alarming fact led to a discussion which revealed that this was the first engagement after a holiday period and obviously the preparation was inadequate.

Another factor becomes clear to every television viewer who watches gymnastics.

In both activities certain joints have to be moved beyond their normal optimal range and the first structures of protection, *i.e.* the ligamentous structures, must therefore be lengthened through training in order to allow the increased movement range. The stretch receptors in this type of formed connective tissue will therefore be stimulated at a later stage, muscle protection therefore is all important in order to prevent injury to joint structure such as cartilage and bony surfaces. If muscles are not strong enough to work under adverse conditions such as cold or inadequate blood supply, tears will easily occur. In dancers the most vulnerable joints are the hip joint, to a certain degree also the joints of the spine. The dancer must be able to perform "the splits" both antero-posteriorly and laterally. In gymnasts the most vulnerable joints are the joints of the lumbar and thoracic regions, to a certain extent also the hip joints. The joints of the vertebral column are already more vulnerable in human beings as they were originally built for a horizontal position of the trunk supported by four uprights. During growth to adult status, this horizontal position has been changed to a vertical position, supported by two uprights. An additional danger is created by the fact that the individual vertebrae are not stacked on top of one another following the line of gravity but the spinal column shows curves in which individual vertebrae are placed in a balanced position anteriorly and posteriorly to the line of gravity. This position must be maintained by muscle power, but gives the trunk an additional quality of elasticity, necessary for other components of the human organism. In modern gymnastics the main axis of movement is transferred into the joint between T12 and Lumbar 1 which combines the main movement elements of the thoracic and lumbar region. This small joint becomes the main axis of movement round which a full jack-knife movement forward and backward can be performed. All this depends on adequate length of ligamentous structures and great muscle power of long and short muscles which can be found anteriorly and posteriorly. The Author has taken the time of the Reader to explain the difficulties under which the movements are performed and how precariously a harmonious interaction of all the structures involved, is balanced.

It also endeavors to stress the fact that no injury of this kind should be treated by a Therapist who has not a basic knowledge of the sport involved. In many cases pain should never be the sole guide to the origin of the injury and the structures involved. Close co-operation between the Trainer and the Therapist is essential.

These injuries are often considered trivial but may incapacitate the patient for a long time. These patients are usually in perfect health and all systems work optimally and *harmoniously.* This state must be preserved as far as possible. I saw recently in a therapeutic journal the suggestion that "chin-ups" were an excellent exercise during the recovery period of an injured runner who had the lower leg in plaster of Paris. I do not wish to enter into any discussion but would like to draw the Reader's attention to the word "harmoniously".

My personal experience is restricted to soft tissue lesions. German Authors (Kohlrausch, Leube) also mention the beneficial effect of C.T.M. in cases of fractures. The areas treated are the areas of more centrally situated areas of vascular anastomosis. A speeding up for the formation of new bone is expected. I wish however to restrict myself to the discussion of soft tissue lesions, based on personal experience or the experience of colleagues. Given the chance I would however consider the use of

C.T.M. in selected fracture cases well worth the effort.

If the treatment of soft tissue lesions is not carefully planned on physiological lines, the injury may recur again at frequent intervals and eventually force the patient to discontinue with their activity. The cause of these injuries is always the use of tissue beyond physiological limits, sometimes also direct trauma, resulting from a collision. The result is a tear or stretch of formed and unformed connective tissue or muscle tissue. As a result of the tear, blood vessels are injured, haemorrhage occurs, exudation of blood and tissue fluid takes place and a haematoma forms. The exudated fluid gradually becomes organised as part of the healing process. Part of it will be reabsorbed, part of it will become organised into scar tissue. It must be realised that muscle tissue cannot be replaced as such. The replacement tissue is always connective tissue in the form of scar tissue, which has a tendency to contract and shorten, very often including some nerve fibres into the scar tissue. Scar tissue is inextensible and if it forms part of a muscular structure a different quotient of expansion is present between the muscle fibres and the scar tissue. Future functional use of the muscle will therefore often cause pain, the muscle will be used incorrectly and future tears often result.

It is therefore essential to plan the treatment on physiological lines. The procedure will depend on the extent of the injury, the principles will always be the same.

The immediate and first approach must be limitation of haemorrhage and exudation. No movement must therefore be allowed which causes further exudation, with the limb at rest various measures are applied to cause vaso-constriction such as ice, sprays of various kinds etc., stitches may be applied, bandages or strapping used. The absorption of exudated fluid must be encouraged as far as possible in order to limit the amount of unavoidable scar tissue. Static hyperaemia as a result of the injury must therefore be changed into active hyperaemia so that inflammatory products can be carried away in the blood and lymphstream. Treatment must also encourage the normal use of the part within physiological limits in order to avoid alienation occurring in the cortical pathway. This is important in order to maintain a certain amount of training during the recovery period and return the athlete to full training as soon as possible. This must however be postponed until the healing process is completed *i.e.* pain free on normal use. To start training too early with the use of painkillers only leads to further injury which eventually forces the athlete to give up the activity.

In order to illustrate the above mentioned principles of treatment, a summary of a frequently occurring injury is given.

The injury concerns the *tear of some fibres of gastrocnemeus*. The sensation described by dozens of patients is almost identical in all cases and leads to an easy diagnosis. While performing activities such as dancing, leaping or playing tennis, the patient feels as if something had hit them suddenly at the back of the leg. I have watched some performers who even turned round in order to find out what was behind them. The rupture of some muscle fibres usually occurs in the lowest fibres of the muscle at the point of their insertion into the soleus tendon. The immediate treatment is to check effusion as described above and prevent weightbearing. To prevent extensive granulation tissue formation the following procedure proved successful:

> The patient is placed in forward lying with the knee in slight flexion, produced by a soft pillow, placed under the lower leg: C.T.M. to the Basic section and the hamstring area. (Both legs.)
>
> Change to lying with the two legs supported in slight elevation: C.T.M. to both thighs, concentrating on the femoral triangle.

In the first described treatment position it is easy to palpate for a comparatively small painful area which represents the area of the actual tear. The patient's leg must not be exposed to gravity before the following strapping is applied: An oval chiropody felt pad, approximately 2½ inches long and 1½ inches wide is placed over the centre of the painful area. Two inch wide non-elastic adhesive strapping is then cut into strips, approximately six inches long, the actual length depends on the circumference of the lower leg. These strips are then applied in a crossed pattern, the crosses running up the centre of the back of the leg, the strips overlapping and running obliquely upward. The first cross starting approximately two inches below the felt pad, continuing upwards to approximately two inches beyond the felt pad. It is essential to provide a gap free of strapping, on the anterior aspect of the leg in order not to interfere with the tibial circulation.The edges of the felt pad should be bevelled to allow the strapping to pass smoothly over it. This makes for even pressure over the injured area. For re-education of walking the patient should wear flat-heeled shoes and heel-toe walking emphasised with free rolling off movement of the foot. It is important that the patient should not walk with a limp so that smooth muscle contraction will act on the circulation. Should walking be too painful on the first day, the patient can be provided with *two* sticks or elbow-crutches. The patient should be treated every day and it is expected that after two days, normal walking is no longer painful with the strapping in position. As long as *pain* persists, the felt pad should be continued under the strapping. The strapping above should be continued for at least another week after all discomfort has disappeared. The above procedure will reduce the scar tissue to a minimum. C.T.M. should be applied every day until all discomfort has disappeared and progressed into the popliteal area but not into the calf. When training is resumed it is advisable to use C.T.M. approximately twice a week before training.

The Author found that this procedure prevents recurrence of this very disabling injury. Reference: Ebner 1965.

CONCLUSIONS

An attempt has been made in the previous chapters to give an introduction to the basis, technique and therapeutic application of connective tissue manipulation. It is important to stress that the technique cannot be learned from the description in a book and that practical instruction is absolutely necessary. Due to the interrelationship of nervous pathways to visceral and somatic structures, correct technique and understanding of the effects of the treatment are important factors in achieving beneficial and not adverse results in the treatment of patients. It is hoped that this book will stimulate interest in this form of treatment which is not intended to replace any proved and valuable form of physiotherapy but may in many cases represent a valuable addition to existing forms of treatment. C.T.M. may represent in some cases the only form of treatment; in others it will be an important adjunct to other therapeutic agents. In the light of the universal inter-relationship of physiological function, it is no longer defensible to ignore this relationship and apply any therapeutic agent in an isolated manner.

The favourable clinical results obtained in this country and abroad are indisputable. A great deal of further information is required as to the mode of action of the manipulation. The author, however, hopes that the information given in this book, inadequate as it is, may stimulate interest into further research. The extensive literature referred to in preparing this book made it abundantly clear how much information is continuously produced in specialized research which is not always correlated for the benefit of the patient.

Future experience may prove that a much wider field of application exists than has been possible to describe in this publication. Recent experience has already widened the field.

REFERENCE

Angevine, D. Murray (1950). *Connective Tissues.* New York: Macy Foundation.

Anning, S. T. (1949). The aetiology of gravitational ulcers of the leg. *Brit. med.J.* **2,** 458.

Appleton, A. B., Hamilton, W. J. & Tchaperoff, I. C. C. (1958). In W. J. Hamilton, and G. Simon, *Surface and Radiological Anatomy for Students and General Practitioners,* 4th ed. Cambridge: Heffer.

Asboe-Hansen, G. (1954). *Connective Tissue in Health and Disease.* Copenhagen: Munksgaard.

Bach, Francis(1950). *Recent Advances in Physical Medicine.* London: Churchill.

Bailey, F.R. (1958). *Bailey's Textbook of Histology,* 12th ed., rev.P. E. Smith and W. M. Copenhaver. London: Baillière, Tindall, & Cox.

Barcroft, H. & Swan, H. J. C. (1953). *Sympathetic Control of Human Blood Vessels.* London: Arnold.

Bartholomew, Audrey, E. *The treatment of Gravitational Ulcers by Physiotherapy.* London: St Thomas' Hospital. The Green Bank Press, London, S.E.1.

Behrend, H. J., M.D. (1954). Further Light on the Rationale of Physical Medicine Procedures. *New York State Journal* Vol. 54 No. 2.

Best, C. H. & Taylor, N. B. (1961). *The Physiological Basis of Medical Practice,* 7th ed. London: Baillière, Tindall & Cox.

Blomfield, L. B. (1950). In *Recent Advances in Physical Medicine,* p. 46, ed. F. Bach. London: Churchill.

Bobath, K. and B. (1975). *Motor Development in the different types of cerebral palsy.*
— B. (1978). *Adult Hemiplegia: Evaluation and Treatment.*
— K. (1980) *A neuro-physiological basis for the treatment of cerebral palsy.*
All available from: Bobath Centre, 5 Netherhall Gardens, Lndon N.W.3.

Chambers, R. & Zweifach, B. W. (1944). Topography and function of the mesenteric capillary circulation. *Amer. J. Anat.* **75,** 173.
— (1947). Intercellular cement and capillary permeability. *Physiol. Rev.* **27,** 436.

Clark, E. R. & Clark, E. L. (1943). Caliber changes in minute blood vessels. Amer. J. Anat. **73,** 215.

Conti, G. (1953). Ueber das Vorkommen von Sperrvorrichtungen in Arterien mit spezieller Beruecksichtigung der "Gestielten Polster." *Acta anat.* **18,** 234.

Cyriax, J. (1950). The treatment of lumber disc lesions. *Brit. Med. J.* **2,** 1434.
— (1953). *Disc Lesions.* London: Cassel.

Dicke, Elisabeth (1953). *Meine Bindegewebsmassage.* Stuttgart: Marquardt.

Dittmar, F. (1943). Die diagnostische und therapeutische Bedeutung der reflektorischen Krankheitszeichen. *Med. Klinik,* **39,** 517.
— (1952). Ueber den Einfluss von Hautreizen und die Funktion innerer Organe. *Z. ges. inn. Med.* **7,** 267.

Ebner, Maria (1956). Peripheral Circulatory Disturbances: Treatment by Massage of Connective Tissue in Reflex Zones. *Brit. J. o. Phys. Med.* Butterworth, London, Vol. 19, No. **8.**

— (1965). Connective Tissue Massage, Application in Migraine and Intermittent Claudication. *South Afr. J. o. Physiotherapy* Vol. XXI, no. **3.**
— Soft Tissue Injuries of Ankle and Calf
— (1968). Connective Tissue Massage, Application to Frozen Shoulder. *New Zealand J. O. Physiotherapy* Vol. 3, No. **14.**

Ebner-Risk (1972). Connective Tissue Massage, Uses and Contra-Indications in Obstetrics and Gynaecology. Newsletter No. **32** *The Obstetric Ass. o. Chartered Physiotherapists.*

Ebner, Maria (1978). Connective Tissue Massage. *"Physiotherapy" Journal o. C. S. P.* July 1978, Vol. **64** No. 7.

Ebner, Maria (1982). A Way to Natural Childbirth. Churchill-Livingstone, Edinburgh.

Freedman, R. R. & Peter Ianni (1983). Role of cold and emotional stress in Raynaud's disease and scleroderma. *B. M. J.* Vol. 287, November 19, 1983.

Fox, R. H. & Hilton, S. M. (1958). Bradykinin formation in human skin as a factor in heat vasodilation. *J. Physiol.* **142,** 219.

Glaeser, O. & Dalicho, A. W. (1955). *Segmentmassage.* Leipzig: Thieme.

Glaeser, W. (1928). Ueber die vasomotorische Innervierung der Blutgefaesse der Milz nebst Bemerkungen zur intermuralen Nervenversorgung der Blutgefaesse im Knochenmark. *Z. Anat. EndwGesch.* **87,** 741.

Grieve, G.P. (1971). The Hip. *Physiotherapy* **57,** 5.
— (1981). *Common Vertebral Joint Problems.* Edinburgh: Churchill-Livingstone.
— (1983) The Hip. *Physiotherapy* **69,**6.

Hafferl, Anton (1953). *Lehrbuch der Topographischen Anatomie.* Berlin: Springer.

Ham, Arthur W. (1957). *Histology,* 3rd ed. London: Lippincott.

Handbuch der Phys. Therapie (1966). Band I
— (1971). Band II, Gustav Fischer Verlag, Stuttgart.

Hansen, K. & von Staa, H. (1938). *Reflektorische und Algetische Krankheitszeichen der Inneren Organe.* Leipzig: Thieme.

Harff, J. (1951). Zur Wirkungsweise der sogenannten Bindegewebsmassage. *Z. Krankengymnast,* **3,** 113.

Hartfall, S. J. (1959). Advances in the treatment of arthritis and chronic rheumatism. *Practitioner,* **183,** 455.

Hartman, F. (1928). Funktionelle Stoerungen der zentralen Kreislauf-organe bei geloester Erkrankung der Koerperdecke. Wien. klin. Schr. **41,** 272.

Head, H. (1898). *Die Sensibilitaetsstoerungen der Haut bei Viszeral Erkrankungen.* Berlin.

Heardman, Helen (1959). *Physiotherapy in Obstetrics and Gynecology,* 2nd ed., rev. M. Ebner. Edinburgh: Livingstone.

Hill, L. C.& Wilson, D. (1950). In *Recent Advances in Physical Medicine,* ed. F. Bck. London: Churchill.

Hilton, S. M. (1959). A peripheral arterial conducting mechanism underlying dilatation of the femoral artery. *J. Physiol.* **149,** 93.

Hudack, S. S. & McMaster, P. D. (1933). The lymphatic participation in human cutaneous phenomena. *J. exp. Med.* **57,** 765.

Iversen, Kurt (1954). Hormonal influence on connective tissue. In *Connective Tissue in Health and Disease,* ed. Asboe-Hansen. Copenhagen: Munksgaard.

Kayser-Petersen, J. E. (1930). *Die Betrachtung und Betastung des Brustkorbes bei Lungenkranken.* Leipzig: Barth.

Knotz, J. (1927). Die Halbseiten-Fernreflexe als diagnostische Wegweiser. *Wien. kline Wschr.* **40,** 1189, 1231.

Kohlrausch,W. (1953). Der Verlauf der reflektorischen Zonen in Haut, Unterhaut und Muskulatur. *Arch. phys. Ther.* **5,** 223.

Landeis, M. E. (1937). Permeability of capillaries. *Harvey Lecture Series,* **32,** p. 70.

Lansing, Albert J. (1959). *The Arterial Wall.* London: Baillière, Tindall & Dox.
Lehrbuch der Physiotherapie (1970). Verlag Volk und Gesundheit, Berlin.

Leube, H. & Dicke, Elisabeth (1948). *Massage Reflextorischer Zonen im Bindegewebe bei Rheumatischen und Inneren Erkrankungen.* Jena* Fischer.

Lewis, Thomas (1927). *The Blood Vessels of the Human Skin and their Responses.* London: Shaw.

Mackenzie (1917). *Krankheitszeichen und ihre Auslegung.* Wuerzburg: Kabitzsch.

McKechnie, A., Wilson, Watson, Scott (1983). Anxiety States:
A Preliminary Report on the Value of Connective Tissue Massage. *J. o. Psychosomatic Research,* Vol. 27, November 2, 1983.

Mennell, J. B. (1945). *Physical Treatment by Movement and Massage.* London: Churchill.

Meyer, Karl (1947). The biological significance of hyaluronic acid and hyaluronidase. *Physiol. Rev.* **27,** 335.

Mitchell, G. A. G. (1953). *Anatomy of the Autonomic Nervous System. 13Edinburgh: Livingstone.*
— (1956). *Cardiovascular Innervation.* Edinburgh: Livingstone.

Montagna, W. (1956). *The Structure and Function of Skin.* New York: Academic Press.

Neuwirth, E., and Gayral, L. (1959) The shoulder-hand syndrome of Barre-Lieou and osteoarthritis of the cervical spine, *Lancet,* Minneapolis **79,** 4 (1960). Current concepts of the cervical portion of the sympathetic nervous system.Lancet, Minneapolis **80,** 7.

Niebauer, G. (1972). Les recepteurs nerveux de la peau. *Kinesetherapie Scientifique* No. 98, December 1972.
— (1977). *Handbuch ueber Klinische Pathologie des vegetativen Nervensystems, Sturm und Birkmayer, Fischer Verlag Stuttgart-New York.*

Nonnenbruch, W. & Gross, D. (1952). Die vasale Ordnung im vegetativen Nervensystem als Grundlage fuer die Neuraltherapy. *Med. Klinik.* 47.

Opperman, H. J. (1949). Ueber vegetative Zeichen bei Erkrankungen des Oberbauches. *Med. Wiss. Ges. Rostock Tag.* **10,**12.

Pullinger, B. D. & Florey, H. W. (1935). Some observations on the structure and functions of lymphatics. *Brit. J. exp. Path.* **16,** 49.

Riley, J. F. (1959). *The Mast Cells.* Edinburgh: Livingstone.

Rouanet, G. (1946). Kapillarmikroskopische Studien bei Erkrankungen innerer Organe. *Dtsch. Ges. Wes.* p. 115.
— (1947). *Z. ges. inn. Med.* p. 151

Schleyer-Saunders, E. (1955). *Backache in Women.* Bristol: Wright.
Symposium on the Functional Implications of Segmental Facilitation. (1955). *J. o. American Osteopathic Ass.* Jan. 1955.

Teirich-Leube, H. (1960). *Grundriss der Bindegewebsmassage.* Stuttgart: Fischer.

Travell, Janet (1951). *Pain Mechanisms in Connective Tissues.* New York: Macy Foundation.

Trueta, J. (1954). Osteoarthritis of the hip. *Ann.R. Coll. Surg. Engl.* **15,** 174.
— (1956). Osteoarthritis. *Lancet,* **1,** 585.

Völker, R. & Rostovsky, E. (1949). Ueber den therapeutischen Wert der B.G.M. bei Gefaess-stoerungen der Gliedmassen. *Z. Rheumaforsch.* **8,** 192.

Walshe, F. M. R. (1958). *Diseases of the Nervous System*, 9th ed. Edinburgh: Livingstone.

Wernoe (1925).*Viscerokutane Reflexe.* Berlin: Springer.

White, J. C. (1954). Conduction of pain in man. *Arch Neurol. Psychiat. Chicago*,**71**,1.

Wilde, F. R. (1951). The perivascular neural pattern of the femoral region. *Brit. J. Surg.* **39**, 97.

Yoffey, J. M. & Courtice, F. C. (1956). *Lymphatics, Lymph andLymphoid Tissue*, 2nd ed. London: Arnold.

Zweifach, B. W. (1954). *The Exchange of Material between Blood Vessels and Lymph Compartments.* New York: Macy Foundation.

INDEX OF CONDITIONS